T0329824

# TRAUMA-SENSITIVE
# YOGA IN THERAPY

# TRAUMA-SENSITIVE
## YOGA IN THERAPY
### Bringing the Body
### Into Treatment

**DAVID EMERSON**

Foreword by Jennifer West, PhD

**W. W. Norton & Company**
New York • London

Note to Readers: Standards of clinical practice and protocol change over time, and no technique or recommendation is guaranteed to be safe or effective in all circumstances. This volume is intended as a general information resource for professionals practicing in the field of psychotherapy and mental health; it is not a substitute for appropriate training, peer review, and/or clinical supervision. Neither the publisher nor the author(s) can guarantee the complete accuracy, efficacy, or appropriateness of any particular recommendation in every respect.

Copyright © 2015 by David Emerson
Foreword copyright © 2015 by Jennifer West, PhD

For information about permission to reproduce
selections from this book, write to Permissions,
W. W. Norton & Company, Inc.,
500 Fifth Avenue, New York, NY 10110

For information about special discounts for bulk purchases, please contact
W. W. Norton Special Sales at specialsales@wwnorton.com or 800-233-4830

Manufacturing by LSC Harrisonburg
Book design by Carole Desnoes
Production manager: Leeann Graham

Library of Congress Cataloging-in-Publication Data

Emerson, David, 1969–
Trauma-sensitive yoga in therapy : bringing the body into treatment /
David Emerson ; foreword by Jennifer West, PhD. — First edition.
     pages cm
"A Norton Professional Book."
Includes bibliographical references and index.
ISBN 978-0-393-70950-6 (hardcover)
1. Psychic trauma—Physical therapy.
2. Yoga—Therapeutic use. I. Title.
RC552.T7E45 2015
616.85'210642—dc23
                                        2014034452

W. W. Norton & Company, Inc.
500 Fifth Avenue, New York, N.Y. 10110
www.wwnorton.com

W. W. Norton & Company Ltd.
15 Carlisle Street, London W1D 3BS

    8 9 0

*To Suzanne Cecilia Dawson Emerson,*
*for the gift of being seen and known.*

# CONTENTS

# ACKNOWLEDGMENTS

I'D LIKE TO THANK MY FAMILY, ESPECIALLY MANDY AND Hazen, for encouraging me to express myself to the best of my abilities. Dad, thanks for your example in general, for pointing out how to be a caring professional and for how to honor and respect the people you actually work for. Thanks to Andrea Costella Dawson and Christine Dahlin at Norton for their unfailing professionalism, their attention to this book, and for their patience with me throughout the writing process. And thanks to all of my clients, colleagues, and students at the Trauma Center and elsewhere, for teaching me how to proceed with integrity—I hope this book honors you all appropriately.

# FOREWORD

Originally, in the first couple sessions, part of me was hyper-
alert of being in the space and distrustful of yoga, ya know,
what is this really going to do for me? I was very skeptical. . . .

[Over time], I know it's kind of strange, but it's almost as if my
mind became more connected to my thoughts and what I did
to my body. . . . [Yoga] gave me structure, like a place to start
building or become more aware. I think it gave me a starting
place.

—Trauma-sensitive yoga research participant

AS A HELPING PROFESSIONAL, EVEN IF YOU HAVE NEVER
used yoga with a client before, you can likely imagine a reaction such as the one depicted above. In fact, you may even
share some of the skepticism described in the first part or
have similar questions about the use of yoga in treatment.
Common questions I have been asked include the following: If other forms of therapy have not successfully eliminated symptoms, how is yoga going to be any different? How
can yoga help in healing the deep wounds of trauma? How can
yoga supplement, or be integrated in, the psychotherapy process? Is yoga a worthy compliment to psychotherapy? By way

of introducing David Emerson's practical and creative ideas on how to integrate yoga into the therapy room, I will attempt to answer these questions and offer my thoughts on how and why yoga is an important and useful adjunct to therapy. My perspective and ideas are based on my clinical experiences and research with adult female survivors of childhood interpersonal trauma, referred to as complex trauma.

My journey into yoga began in 2004 after a significant personal loss. Practicing yoga became a source of hope and healing during a time of turmoil. Like many of the clients I now work with, I found a physical, psychological, and emotional outlet through yoga, and my personal journey quickly became an integral part of my professional practice. As a counseling psychologist who studies posttrauma recovery and healing, I always look for ways to help my clients decrease symptoms and improve overall health and wellness. After noticing yoga's profound effects on my own emotional well-being and recovery, I began to wonder how people struggling with complex trauma might respond to yoga. Indeed, a growing body of literature has unequivocally shown the benefits of yoga for many medical problems (e.g., diabetes, arthritis, fibromyalgia, cancer) and mental health issues (e.g., depression, anxiety), so it seemed reasonable to imagine possible benefits for trauma survivors.

As I ventured toward using yoga as a therapeutic outlet, I took yoga teacher training to educate myself further and began researching yoga as a treatment for posttraumatic stress disorder (PTSD).. In collaboration with Bessel van der Kolk's Trauma Center, I focused my research on examining the effects of TSY) on adult survivors of complex trauma.

What we know about complex trauma is that the symptoms that arise in the aftermath can disrupt functioning well into adulthood and pervade all domains of a person's life. When our self-protective capacities are consistently overwhelmed by repeated exposure to trauma it can be toxic to our bodies, and survivors often find themselves in a cycle of hyperarousal and dissociative numbing. The experience of complex trauma and resulting autonomic instability can lead to a feeling of being out of control within one's own body and life. Trauma survivors describe intolerable physical sensations and somatic complaints, problems with affect and impulse regulation, deficits in attentional capacities, poor interoceptive awareness, and negative self-perception.

This complex array of symptoms can pose significant challenges in treatment. After all, how can we expect clients to successfully engage in talk therapy when they disconnect from inner experiences, struggle to stay connected to their present experiences, and lack the skills to tolerate affect elicited by trauma-related stimuli, such as when asked to process traumatic memories? Psychotherapy can be effective in treating various aspects of PTSD, such as confronting relational difficulties in a supportive environment, identifying unhealthy patterns, and setting goals for engaging in self-care. However, physiological symptoms, somatic complaints, and a lack of interoceptive awareness may be more difficult to treat with "top-down approaches" (i.e., cognitively oriented treatments focusing on thoughts and emotions). This leads us back to the question about how yoga can help.

## How is yoga going to be any different from other treatments?

Yoga—defined here as a combination of physical forms, focused breathing, and purposeful attention or mindfulness—seems to be a useful complement to trauma treatment because it directly targets the very symptoms that other approaches struggle to address by using the body purposefully (i.e., a bottom-up approach). TSY in particular aims to cultivate awareness of the mind-body connection and to build self-regulation skills to address the ways in which trauma is held in the body.

A randomized controlled trial (RCT), conducted by Bessel van der Kolk and colleagues (van der Kolk et al., 2014), examined the effects of TSY on women with complex trauma who were unresponsive to traditional psychotherapy. Women in the 10-week TSY course were more likely than women in the control group to no longer meet criteria for PTSD posttreatment. The TSY group also showed significant decreases in depressive symptoms and negative tension- reduction behaviors (e.g., self-injury). Furthermore, a long-term follow-up conducted by Alison Rhodes (2014) found that the frequency of continuing yoga practice, regardless of group assignment in the study, was a significant predictor of long-term outcomes. At 1 to 3 years posttreatment, women who practiced yoga following the study were more likely to show a loss of a PTSD diagnosis and greater reductions in PTSD and depressive symptoms (Rhodes, 2014). These studies suggest that the addition of TSY to treatment may lead to long-term improvement in symptoms that had previously been considered unresponsive to other interventions.

# How can yoga help to heal the deep wounds of trauma?

While past research has demonstrated the profound effects of TSY as an effective complement to traditional psychotherapy, the specific mechanisms by which TSY generates such change were still unclear. In an attempt to gain some understanding, I talked with participants 2 months after they completed the 10 weeks of TSY. Using semistructured interviews in a one-on-one setting, I asked the women to share their personal experiences of TSY and the perceived changes in their lives due to their use of TSY.

Throughout the interviews, the women attested to the tenaciousness of complex trauma symptoms and their nonresponsiveness to years of treatment. Through their experiences with TSY, they reported symptom reduction, improved quality of life, and personal empowerment. Through the sharing of their stories, the women provide some answers to this question about how yoga can help in healing the deep wounds of trauma. I outline some of their insights below.

Consistent with typical symptoms of complex trauma, participants in the study described how, prior to the TSY program, they often felt disconnected or dissociated from their present reality. However, the integration of purposeful attention with physical postures and focused breathing seemed to improve participants' capacity for present-moment awareness. They became increasingly able and willing to notice how they were feeling in their body and formed greater tolerance for emotional states and bodily sensations, as they could experience them in a safe way, rather than from the lens of past trauma. One participant said she "started to be able to recognize emotions . . . feel what's inside . . . instead of just trying to get rid of it."

In addition to greater interoceptive awareness and tolerance of inner sensations, TSY also instilled a sense of ownership over one's physical body that many women had lost through their traumatic experiences. Women started to recognize that their bodies belong to them, that their bodies were under their control, and that they could be safe in their bodies. This involved a literal awareness of an embodied self, an acceptance of one's body with less judgment and criticism, as well as a sense of being in charge of how to move, use, and treat one's body. For many of the participants, a growing awareness of ownership and control over one's body also led to appreciation for one's body, including a deeper sense of responsibility for self-care and the tendency to "listen to [my body] a lot more now." Similarly, participants said they began to feel more confident in identifying and employing appropriate behavioral responses in emotionally difficult situations, including when they triggered or experienced flashbacks. Through TSY they were able to build skills for emotion regulation through the use of physical postures and breath, and "have these ways to soothe and comfort myself, and I don't have to be stuck in the flashbacks."

The increased ability for regulation of internal states also inspired a sense of control in one's life and, in turn, hopes for new possibilities in the future. For some, this included willingness to take action to improve their health (e.g., stop smoking or drinking) and for others this consisted of making changes to improve quality of life (e.g., pursuing professional passions).

Like many survivors of complex trauma, the women also experienced long-lasting damage to their sense of self, such as feelings of shame, hopelessness, and worthlessness. However, through TSY, participants began to change their language about themselves, express less self-judgment, and even cultivate self-acceptance. Likewise, participants acknowledged an appreciation for all they had been through.

Issues of interpersonal functioning (e.g., isolation, lack of trust, unhealthy boundaries) resulting from complex trauma caused some of the most significant pain for participants. However, as participants began to feel more connected to, and accepting of, themselves they also began feeling more comfortable engaging authentically in relationships and setting healthy boundaries.

While the TSY classes focused specifically on present-moment experiences in the body, the women in the study described benefits both on and off the mat. The women gained skills for finding a calm presence in and out of class, they developed a stronger connection to themselves and to other people in their lives, and they recognized their ability to choose how to move their bodies and choose the direction of their lives.

## How can TSY supplement, or be integrated in, the psychotherapy process?

The impact of TSY on trauma survivors can clearly be quite significant. Ideally, the integration of TSY with ongoing psychotherapy would allow for the synthesis of top-down and bottom-up processing in the treatment setting. Such an approach rests on the belief that a greater capacity for emotion regulation, interoceptive awareness, and self-acceptance may facilitate deeper interpersonal connections (including the therapy relationship). Indeed, some participants expressed greater ability for emotional expression and exploration in therapy for these reasons.

Integrating TSY into the therapy room may seem daunting at first. You may wonder about space limitations or whether clients will feel comfortable doing yoga forms in the therapy room. While this book will walk you through all the ins and outs and address these curiosities in detail, here are some brief thoughts regarding such concerns.

From a practical standpoint, many of the movements and forms in TSY are done in a chair, making this approach easily adaptable to the individual therapy room. The information contained in this book will provide you with many examples. Additionally, some of the study participants offered insight into specific attributes of the teacher and environment that made them feel comfortable and able to fully engage in moving their bodies in a therapeutic setting. I would suggest that these characteristics (outlined below) would also be important for a therapist in a clinical setting.

The tone of the teacher's voice as well as the words the teacher chose were quite important to the facilitation of a sense of safety and comfort. More specifically, a gentle tone and environment of acceptance was appreciated as the teacher was perceived as "extraordinarily kind and patient" and never asked the women to "do more than we could."

Another important aspect was the use of invitatory language (e.g., "if you like" or "when you feel ready"), which highlights choice, presence, and awareness of the body. Furthermore, providing verbal modifications and alternative forms was an important facet to emphasizing choice and reminding the women to pay attention to what feels right in their body. Using invitatory language and emphasizing choice are often helpful in a psychotherapy setting, and this is certainly the case when incorporating TSY. This may be particularly important if and when a client is not ready to verbally address trauma-related material, as we can offer helpful alternatives and "'meet clients where they are.'"

A sense of safety in the room was another critical aspect as it allowed participants to more easily remain engaged in the TSY classes. For example, most participants were grateful for the lights being on, the private room, and the focus on verbal assists versus physical assists. Given the boundaries typically adhered to in therapy, these are likely good guidelines for a psychotherapy setting as well.

## Is yoga a worthy complement to psychotherapy?

The information shared above reflects the valuable role that TSY may have in the treatment of complex trauma. The focus on bottom-up processing in TSY and the emphasis on movement, breath, and bodily sensations seem to help survivors learn to regulate affective arousal by raising awareness of internal states and reorganizing the physiological responses connected to symptoms. Survivors are then more able to experience emotions safely in the present moment.

Whereas recalling the trauma may have elicited reactions such as hyperarousal or dissociation in the past, with these physiological changes and skills for self-regulation, participants are able to manage the trauma-related physical sensations or feelings as they arise. Furthermore, for a number of participants, a greater ability to tolerate trauma-related stimuli also meant greater ease in verbally expressing and processing their experiences in psychotherapy.

While complex trauma has posed some very difficult challenges for treatment, TSY offers an additional approach for working with symptoms of complex trauma and creates new pathways for healing and personal growth. I hope that this book offers hope and inspiration to you. Remember that yoga is a practice of living the process, and David Emerson is a wonderful guide to have on this journey. Enjoy. You are in good hands.

—Jennifer West, PhD

# INTRODUCTION

AT THIS POINT IN HISTORY, THANKS TO THE WORK OF MANY
great practitioners and scientists, we have collectively developed a solid understanding about how traumatic experiences
affect human beings. The picture developed by such lumi-
naries as John Eric Erichsen, Jean-Martin Charcot, Pierre
Janet, John Bowlby, Mary Ainsworth, Lenore Terr, Judith
Herman, Rachel Yehuda, Bessel van der Kolk, and many
other pioneers reveals the devastating impacts of trauma
on our minds, our bodies, and our relationships. Thanks to
continued research in such fields as human development,
neurobiology, and epigenetics, our understanding of trauma
and its impacts continues to deepen and expand. However,
because of the degree of suffering that trauma represents
in human terms, from survivors of war, violence, torture,
human trafficking, and terror to survivors of chronic childhood abuse and neglect to victims of domestic violence and
sexual assault all across the globe, the time has come for us
to pivot from our understanding of trauma toward developing and implementing new, effective treatments. Too many
studies that indicate the impacts of trauma tend to resort to

the hope of a psychopharmacological solution; while perhaps drugs can take the edge off of symptoms (and may even one day erase memories), it is extremely doubtful that they will ever truly heal people from the most insidious reality of relational trauma: that we were deliberately hurt and betrayed by our fellow human beings (most egregiously, by those who were supposed to protect us). TSY is intended most pointedly for people who have experienced this kind of interpersonal trauma and, though I allude to it here, I will explain the rationale in detail.

My basic argument throughout this book is that if we want to treat people who have experienced interpersonal trauma effectively we must use the clinical knowledge available to us and be open to new interventions that recognize the deep and complex nature of these traumatic experiences and not reduce trauma to a set of symptoms that can be medicated away, or for which a simple change in cognitive frame or behavioral patterns will suffice. Our treatments must match the complexity and nuance of trauma itself, and one aspect of the whole person that must not be overlooked or minimized is the experience of being embodied. For it is the body, the result of billions of years of evolution, that ultimately defines us as being human.

In this book I explain the fundamentals of trauma-sensitive yoga (TSY), an intervention based in and completely reliant on the body, as an adjunctive treatment for individuals impacted by trauma. My intention is to offer a rationale for its use, describe the evidence accumulated on its behalf so far, and provide specific techniques and practices that can be utilized by clinicians and clients as they work together to heal one of the most insidious wounds a human being can experience.

In 2003 yoga was first used as an adjunctive treatment for trauma at the Trauma Center in Brookline, Massachusetts. From its beginning, the Trauma Center Yoga Program has been a collaborative effort among yoga teachers, clinicians, neuroscientists, and our clients. In keeping with our desire to accumulate objective data as to the efficacy of our intervention, one of the first steps we took was to create a small pilot study to measure in a clinical setting the impact of yoga on adult survivors of chronic childhood abuse and neglect. Our concern was that our clients as a group reported explicitly or demonstrated in various ways a deep and abiding hatred for their bodies, and we did not see a talk-based approach to therapy as being an adequate way to engage such visceral self-hatred. We thought we could use yoga as a way to help people to befriend their bodies and that this newfound friendliness would contribute to positive therapeutic outcomes. Therefore, as a team, the first measurement we came up with was a body awareness scale that we could use to measure trauma sufferers' sense of themselves and relationship to their physical beings. This instrument was proprietary so it had never been used or tested in any other study, but we wanted to see if doing yoga could indeed change a traumatized person's perceptions of her body. In addition we decided to compare our yoga group to a dialectical behavior therapy (DBT) group that was ongoing in our clinic. We chose DBT for comparison because it is a treatment often used for trauma survivors and it is primarily a cognitive approach as opposed to our use of yoga, which is primarily physical. I should say that, at this point in our work, we referred to our intervention simply as "yoga" or "gentle yoga." It wasn't until we really started to establish the theoretical underpinnings and specific methodology behind our approach that we coined the specific term trauma-sensitive yoga.

What did we learn as a result of this simple survey and comparison? The yoga group did indeed feel much better about their bodies, and the DBT group felt the same or worse about theirs (van der Kolk, 2006). This simple result in our small pilot study encouraged us to look further into the possibilities of yoga as a beneficial intervention within the context of trauma treatment.

After a few years we were able to conduct another, slightly larger pilot study that was also positive in terms of body perception, this time comparing our group of trauma survivors with a group without a significant trauma history. Then, in 2009, we were fortunate enough to receive the first grant ever awarded by the National Institutes of Health (NIH) to study the use of yoga for trauma. For the purposes of this study, in order to generate some empirically sound data, we needed to study the effects of our yoga protocol on symptoms associated with posttraumatic stress disorder (PTSD). In this book I discuss some of the differences between PTSD and other trauma frameworks that, while not officially diagnostic at the time of this writing, nonetheless, more accurately describe the clients for which TSY was developed. These phenomena include complex posttraumatic stress disorder (CPTSD), complex trauma, and developmental trauma, all of which imply a more prolonged exposure to interpersonal trauma, such as a child growing up in an abusive home, as opposed to a single incident, like a car accident, which might result in a PTSD diagnosis. So, while the subjects in our study were survivors of multiple, interpersonal traumas, usually beginning in early childhood, everyone also had to qualify for a PTSD diagnosis in order for us to be able to measure any clinically relevant changes that might result after 10 weeks of TSY. Our hypothesis was that TSY participants would show a clinically significant reduction in PTSD symptomology and this is, in fact, what we found (van der Kolk et al., 2014). As a result we are now able to say that TSY is a promising intervention that has clinical relevance for people in treatment for PTSD.

However, as I indicated, there is more to the story because our study also included in-depth interviews with TSY participants that were intended to address the deeper meaning of the TSY experience in relation to the impacts of the complex, long-term, interpersonal trauma that our study subjects had experienced. These qualitative interviews, designed and implemented by Jennifer West (West, 2011) and written about by her in the foreword to this book, indeed revealed a more complex picture. PTSD symptoms in particular were positively affected after 10 weeks of TSY and participants also reported that the TSY practice had an impact on their lives beyond the PTSD symptom set; that is, not just symptoms were affected but also participants experienced themselves in the world and in relation to other people in profoundly new ways.

So we concluded that TSY is a relevant intervention for people with PTSD who also have complex trauma histories.

This indication, which was revealed in our clinical trials, also aligns with our personal experience of using TSY with complexly traumatized individuals, both male and female, youths and adults, in a wide variety of settings. As a result of our clinical trials, the Trauma Center Yoga Program developed a team of qualified yoga teachers who have collectively taught thousands of TSY sessions since 2003 to groups and individuals suffering from complex trauma, including men and women who grew up in abusive or neglectful environments, as well as survivors of interpersonal violence, sexual assault, war, torture, and more. Over the course of this book, I will share examples of some of these stories with you (please note that all names used in the stories throughout are pseudonyms, and all of the case stories are composites based on clinical experiences). Ultimately, this book is intended to equip you with information and techniques that you can use in your therapy work; it should not simply serve as an interesting read, though I hope it is that as well.

I begin in Chapter 1 by exploring the principles and parameters of TSY, including how it differs from traditional yoga and other somatic (or body-based) models of therapy; what its theoretical underpinnings are; which clients can benefit from it most; and who might not be best suited to take advantage of the therapeutic qualities of TSY.

The remaining chapters highlight the core aspects of TSY methodology. I will introduce the key concepts of interoception, choice making, and action taking, and I examine how to use TSY for such therapeutic goals as working with rhythm and movement, being present, and sensing muscle dynamics. Throughout, I offer a look at both why and how to use various aspects of the treatment under different conditions and with different clients, in order to maximize the results. While by no means being exhaustive, the book will end with a "portfolio" chapter that presents a number of illustrated yoga forms that readers can use as soon as they and their clients feel ready to do so.

Before we delve into the rest of the book, I'd like to highlight an important, foundational concept of TSY: you do not need to be a yoga teacher, or really have any prior experience with yoga for that matter, in order to incorporate TSY into your practice. In fact, this book assumes that most readers are not yoga teachers but are approaching the material as qualified mental health clinicians or the equivalent. You will rely first and foremost on your clinical training in order to help you establish when TSY might be appropriate for a given client and then to be able to titrate its use, depending on your assessment of its efficacy. That said, the more familiarity you develop with the contents of this book and with specific TSY practices, the more integrity the intervention will have. My assumption is that if you conclude TSY is good for your client you will also notice that in many fundamental ways it is also good for you so you will be interested in practicing it for yourself, and thereby strengthen your effectiveness as a facilitator!

My hope is that this book, while providing some insight into the nature and impacts of trauma exposure, will be a useful guide to a new treatment modality that has the potential to increase the benefits of your clinical work.

# Interlude

> When the truth is finally recognized, survivors can begin their
> recovery.                                        —Judith Herman, M.D.

> Historical truth is established by what gets told, not by what
> actually happened.                                —Daniel N. Stern

Judith Herman, a pioneer in the field of modern trauma study
and treatment, suggests that "when the truth is finally recognized, survivors can begin their recovery." But what does it
mean to "recognize truth"? What is truth? It may be that the
truth Dr. Herman is pointing to here is what one remembers
about the past. Indeed, many trauma-informed therapists
believe that it is critical for survivors to have access to this
kind of truth: that which we remember. However, Daniel N.
Stern, a pioneer in the field of developmental psychology, an
expert in infant development, and the author of the book
The Interpersonal World of the Infant, says that the "historical truth is established by what gets told, not by what actually happened." Now we have to consider our relationship to
the truth: is it something we know or is it something we tell?
In fact, with trauma, there has historically existed a tension
between what actually happened and what is told about it.
One way to resolve this tension would be to decide what is
more important: what is told or what actually happened. TSY
was developed in a context where what actually happened
matters more than what is told about it. Further, the truth of
"what actually happened," which Stern calls our attention to,
may not be something carried in our explicit memory and

therefore may not be something we can either fully recall or tell someone else about. It may be something that only our body knows and remembers. In fact, it may be something that we cannot speak of but that we can feel with great clarity right now in our bodies: the eloquence of what we feel but cannot tell. So the truth of memory and cognition is not the only kind of truth that is important to trauma healing. What I feel in my body right now, in the present moment, is at least as important as what I remember about the past and what I tell about it.

This book demonstrates that it would be equally valid in the context of trauma treatment to say that, when the truth is finally felt and acknowledged in the body, survivors can begin their recovery.

# TRAUMA-SENSITIVE
# YOGA IN THERAPY

# 1

# WHAT IS TRAUMA-SENSITIVE YOGA?

THIS CHAPTER WILL INTRODUCE TRAUMA-SENSITIVE YOGA (TSY) as a clinical intervention. In order to give as full a picture as possible, I will explore both how TSY differs from mainstream yoga and other somatic models of trauma treatment as well as the theoretical underpinnings of TSY within which I provide an overview of the condition that it is intended to treat (called complex trauma). In order to define complex trauma, I will need to review some of the clinical work that has led to the specific framework as well as some other pertinent clinical material. My presentation of the clinical material is by no means intended to be a complete survey of the literature on trauma. Readers interested in more in-depth works on the subject will find a good place to start within the references section. In defining complex trauma, I begin at a very particular historical point and focus only on what has led me to develop this approach to treatment.

Let's begin by investigating some ways in which TSY differs from more mainstream yoga.

## How does TSY differ from regular yoga?

Yoga is composed of a vast multitude of practices that have a rich, complex, and ancient history. Because yoga as a phenomenon is so convoluted it would be folly to attempt a concise definition. It is more accurate to say that yoga is supple enough to be many different things to many different people. However, in an effort to find a common denominator, I would suggest that people practice yoga because they want to live more fully. Yoga practitioners are curious about the potential that being alive affords them. So whether the practices are more mystical and esoteric in nature or are more grounded and physical, those who take up a yoga practice, whether they are seekers in ancient India or young women in modern-day New York City, share a common bond, which is to know more about themselves and about what it means to be human. Because it is well outside of the scope of this book to go into the historical record in any detail, readers who are interested can find many great resources that investigate the origins and philosophy of yoga as it has existed and evolved over the millennia (one place to start is Feuerstein, 1998).

So, while we have narrowed a definition of yoga down to practices undertaken through a desire to live life more fully, we must next consider the current historical period and how yoga has generally come to be practiced. In that regard, as of the writing of this book, yoga is primarily practiced as a physical discipline that utilizes various body forms in order to strengthen and stretch muscles. In addition to the physical emphasis, other common aspects of yoga in its current iteration are breathing practices and, one of the key buzzwords of our time, mindfulness, which is essentially synonymous with purposeful attention (more on this in Chapter 2). TSY borrows from all of these components: there is an overarching implication that people engaged in TSY want more from life than is currently available to them; we focus on physical forms; we use some simple breathing practices; and we purposefully direct our attention. In these ways TSY is similar to most yoga classes that exist today. However, it is not primarily the external characteristics that distinguish TSY from other types of yoga (though there are a few worth examining), but rather how the material is presented; whether or not yoga becomes a treatment for complex trauma hinges on the presentation.

While the bulk of this book focuses on how to present yoga so that it can become a treatment for complex trauma, let's begin by looking at some general principles of TSY that make it distinct. I will present these principles in contrast to what is typical in what I call a "regular" yoga class, which is my shorthand for a yoga class you are most likely to find in an average Western city. I do recognize that in reality not all yoga classes are the same. Along with the way that forms, breath, and mindfulness are presented in regular yoga versus TSY, I will also consider how language is used in both contexts.

## Forms

In most regular yoga classes the term "pose" is used to refer to each of the postural exercises: that is, Tree Pose, Happy Baby Pose, Eagle Pose, and so on. Because we work with many people who have been made to literally pose for an abuser in either a sexual or exploitative way we realized we had to find another term. Even for our clients who have not experienced sexual exploitation, like some of our war veterans, the term "pose" implies an externalization of the process that implies that what we are doing is more about what it looks like from the outside rather than what it feels like. For these reasons in particular we settled on the term "form" to describe the postural exercises so I use this term going forward.

While TSY uses yoga forms that may show up in any yoga class anywhere, the emphasis is not on the form itself. That is, the focus is not on the external expression of the form but rather on the internal experience of the practitioner. There is no emphasis on "getting a form right" or on pleasing some external authority (namely, the yoga teacher or the clinician). The focus is instead on the practitioners' experiences with the given form as they perceive it. This kind of orientation, from the external to the internal, is one of the key shifts that makes TSY a treatment for complex trauma, and we will come back to this in many ways throughout the book. By valuing the internal perspective over the external in everything we do and say, we send a clear message about power dynamics: with TSY, power resides within the subjective purview of each individual and is not externalized or centralized in the teacher.

So we experiment with different ways of moving our bodies and different shapes that our bodies can make but only so that we have an opportunity to feel something, not so that we can try to mold ourselves to someone else's idea of a form.

The form-based, or body-based, quality of TSY is, however, critically important to the whole project. I would speculate that it is the very fact that we are always working within the context of a yoga form, something visceral and body-based and not in the context of cognition, that gives TSY its particular value as part of the therapeutic process for trauma survivors. For example, imagine that your client tells you that for the past several months when she had her lunch break during work she couldn't feel whether or not she was hungry and this has caused her a great deal of anxiety. Furthermore, your client might tell you that her consternation around food reminds her of never having enough to eat as a child. It would be possible to spend the therapy session talking about that past experience, trying to make sense out of it in some way. It would also be possible to use the therapy session to plan for what to do the next time she has a lunch break and can't feel whether or not she is hungry. A third option would be to spend the session talking about the meaning of food for your client and wondering if perhaps the idea of nourishment is a fundamental traumatic experience. Each of these possibilities may have therapeutic value but they are all indisputably abstract, theoretical, cognition-based exercises: contemplating the past, planning for the future, or trying to create meaning, in this case connecting an inability to recognize what kind of food would be satiating to past trauma.

TSY offers another possibility that also addresses some core issues but in a different way. The client and therapist might employ part of the session to experiment with using a yoga form to practice feeling something like having feet on the ground or contracting or lengthening a muscle. While your client may have told you about her distress at not being able to feel hunger with TSY you and your client will get to practice feeling something in the body right in the moment and choosing what to do about it in real time. In order for this kind of intervention or practice to make sense, we need to understand the problem as one of not being able to feel *any* internal state and not just specifically hunger. If that is the case, we can use a yoga form to practice feeling and choosing what to do in the body with the understanding that it might impact the very same mechanisms that allow us to feel and respond to hunger. In fact, in our experience with TSY at the Trauma Center, feeling a muscle do something is as valid and equally as important as feeling hunger.

I explore this idea in more detail in Chapter 2 but for now we are recognizing that the forms themselves are not important but rather it is the opportunities they offer to have felt experiences in our body that make forms meaningful in the context of TSY. In most regular yoga classes there are goals related to the forms themselves, like holding a form longer or stretching further or making your body conform more fully to the teacher's ideal.

### Breath

In TSY, we experiment with breath but we do not prescribe a way to breathe. In other words, the facilitator does not assume that one way of breathing is inherently better than another way of breathing and, therefore, does not present the material that way. In most regular yoga classes, breath is highly prescriptive, where one way of breathing is presented as "better" than another and the goal is to breathe in the "better" way. For example, it is common to go to a yoga class and hear the teacher say something like, "Extend your out breath; this will help you stay calm." Therefore, it is clear to the student that a long out breath is better than a short one. Once a clinician at the Trauma Center was doing TSY with a war veteran and he invited him to try to extend his out breath a little bit. The veteran became very upset and said that, in the Marines, you were taught to pull the trigger of your gun on the out breath. He was a sniper and had killed many people on an out breath. In this case, simply exhaling for a longer period was not calming or soothing, no matter what the yoga teacher (or clinician) says. For this veteran, a long exhale caused him a great deal of anxiety. For us this was an important lesson in complex trauma treatment: the client's subjective experience is more important than any external idea of how the practice is or "should be." Breath, like form, is presented as an opportunity to experiment with options without any coercion or expectation of outcome (more on breath in Chapters 6 and 7).

## Mindfulness

One simple definition of mindfulness is that it is the purposeful direction of attention toward an object (i.e., a sound, a smell, a taste, an emotion, or a body experience). Jon Kabat-Zinn, a modern proponent and popularizer of mindfulness, says, "Mindfulness means paying attention in a particular way: on purpose, in the present moment, and nonjudgmentally" (Kabat-Zinn, 1994, p.4). When mindfulness comes up in a regular yoga class, it could be anything from paying attention to what you are doing with your body to what you are thinking or what kinds of emotions are coming up.

In TSY we also experiment with the purposeful direction of attention but the object of mindfulness is always the same: the body experience. We are not interested in any other objects: not thoughts, feelings, emotions, sights, sounds, or smells. With TSY, any time the facilitator invites the direction of attention, it is toward what is felt in the body. There is a word for this kind of attention to felt experience in the body that is probably the single most important word in this entire book: interoception. There will be much more on this in the next chapter and the chapters that follow but, for now, please consider that when we talk about mindfulness in TSY it is always connected to interoception.

### Language

The language of the TSY facilitator is critically important and must be chosen with great care and precision. In most regular yoga classes it is common to hear the frequent use of instructions or commands like "raise your right arm" or "place your right foot forward and your left foot back." With TSY we never speak in commands and instead shift entirely to what we call invitatory language. Invitatory language requires that everything you do with TSY is an invitation to your client, including whether or not they do any yoga at all! So "would you like to try a little bit of yoga?" would be an appropriate way to introduce TSY. Then you need to respond to your client's choice: yes or no. They may very well say, "I don't know," because not knowing what to do with the body is a common phenomenon with complex trauma as we will see. In that case you could offer to look at this book together or give them a chapter or two to take home and read if they are interested. The key point is that nothing you do with TSY is a command.

Once you get into the forms themselves, the encouragement for the facilitator is to precede every cue with an invitatory phrase such as "if you like" or "when you are ready." For example, "If you like, you could experiment with lifting one leg" or "When you are ready, you may wish to experiment with lifting your arms." When presented in this way, every action becomes an opportunity for the student to ask herself, "Do I want to lift my leg?" or "Am I ready to lift my arms?" Maybe she decides she is not ready to lift her arms and she pauses for a moment. For traumatized people who may not be used to making these kinds of decisions about what to do with their bodies, invitatory language may be very difficult to deal with because they may not know what they want to do; this is very common. But giving your clients real invitations and allowing them opportunities to consider what they want to do and when they want to do it are also key parts of the treatment.

When you set this kind of invitatory tone and stick with it, your client will learn that he is in charge of what he does with his body. This includes the fact that he can always stop doing TSY at any time for any reason (you can remind him of this possibility). You are not telling your client what to do with his body: he is figuring it out for himself with your support. If you, as the TSY facilitator, notice that your client is becoming frustrated or upset in some way by the practice (or he tells you so) perhaps ask if he would like to stop the practice for now so that he has a chance to decide for himself. He is still able to keep that element of control though you may offer options. The encouragement is that once you introduce TSY everything that your client does with his body is invitational and under his control.

## How TSY differs from other somatic models

Now that we have defined some ways in which TSY differs from regular yoga practice, I would like to shift toward the clinical domain and explain how TSY fits in among other body-based interventions for trauma that have arisen over the past few decades. Though the field of trauma treatment is still primarily anchored in the psychodynamic, psychotherapeutic model that emphasizes cognition (that is, centered on what is spoken between the therapist and client and on helping clients expose and change what are perceived as faulty thought patterns), somatic interventions have become more prominent. By "somatic" I mean any clinical intervention that includes, indicates, or acknowledges the body in some way. Because some of the more elegantly conceived somatic techniques are used exclusively for the alleviation of physical pain (like the work of Thomas Hanna) and others (like the work of Don Hanlon Johnson) are so broad and far-reaching that they don't articulate specific technique but rather act as a more descriptive paradigm for an entire field called "somatics," I will focus on only three widely known interventions that contain within their framework specific techniques that are intended to be utilized in the treatment of psychological trauma.

**The Hakomi method.** Described primarily as a mindfulness practice by its founder, Ron Kurtz, this method also undeniably works with the body (Kurtz, 1990). Kurtz describes how a client will often exhibit a physical gesture in connection with an emotion like lifting the shoulders when afraid. He refers to these physical gestures that accompany emotion as "spontaneous management behavior." From Kurtz's perspective, spontaneous management behavior is not something to judge or even to change but rather something to notice, something to make conscious and even embrace. Though TSY shares aspects of this nonjudgmental awareness, our focus is on the body and not on any meaning making associated with the body experience.

**Sensorimotor psychotherapy.** Its founder, Pat Ogden, describes sensorimotor psychotherapy as "body oriented talk therapy." Ogden has a background in yoga and dance, and she brought that sensibility to her clinical work with trauma survivors. Like the Hakomi method (Ogden was a cofounder with Ron Kurtz of the Hakomi Institute in 1981), a significant amount of time is devoted to working with the physical representation of emotional experiences: how the body contains and expresses emotional valence associated with trauma and how we can use the body to mediate that emotional suffering through the guidance of a qualified clinician (Ogden, Minton, & Pain, 2006).

**Somatic experiencing (SE).** Its founder, Peter Levine, describes SE as having evolved from his observations of prey animals who, in his estimation, though they are chronically exposed to stress, rarely exhibit symptoms of trauma. He believes that prey animals literally use their bodies to move the stress out of their system through actions like shaking. Levine believes that many traumatized people, though in possession of the same physical resources that prey animals have, are, for whatever reason, not able to access them, and therefore the trauma remains stuck physically in the organism. The intention of SE is to help clients gain access to the healing potential inherent in their bodies. SE, like TSY, does not require people to talk about their trauma and relies heavily on the body to facilitate healing (Levine, 1997).

Each of these somatic or body-conscious techniques, to one degree or another, considers the body experience of the client to contain information that is useful to the therapeutic process and makes an attempt to access that information. Whether a matter of identifying and acting out physical gestures that have heretofore been stuck in the body, unable to be expressed (as in Pat Ogden's work), or figuring out ways the body can move to release the imprint that trauma has left on the nervous system (as in Peter Levine's work), clearly the body is central to these therapeutic techniques.

Because of the centrality of the body in the process, TSY is part of what I would call the somatic movement in trauma treatment. However, it is useful to draw some distinctions between these other somatic approaches to trauma treatment and TSY. In my opinion, all three of the methods indicated above attempt, ultimately, to make meaning out of body experiences or to place body experiences in the context of memories or experiences from that past that remain in some way unprocessed. When we talk about memory in the context of trauma, it is often more appropriate to discuss emotion. In other words, Kurtz, Ogden, and Levine all suggest that traumatic memory is primarily encoded as emotion and that these emotions are mediated by the body. In this way, body experiences are important because of their connection to emotional content, and the treatment, in all three cases, is mostly about using your body to change your relationship to emotions: I do something with my body in order to express or relieve emotional content. Importantly, the three methods named above were founded by people trained in Western psychotherapy or psychology, which has an unyielding emphasis on the preeminence of cognition: if I can recognize my emotional state, I can have control over it and if I have some control over it I won't suffer. In other words, these treatments access the body, not as an end in and of itself but rather as a doorway to a cognitive understanding of the emotional valence associated with trauma. This is not to say that these somatic methods are not incredibly beneficial. They have made great contributions to the work of trauma treatment and healing. However, they are ultimately meaning-making paradigms: I shrug my shoulders because I am scared; I want to hit you because I never hit my perpetrator and that act of not hitting is stuck in my body; my back is tight because I have not released the traumatic memory that is stuck there. Other than sharing a focus on the body as part of treatment, TSY is fundamentally different.

In TSY there is no attempt to make meaning out of a body experience; we are not interested in the emotional content associated with a bodily form. In other words, there is no "because" (as in *I shrug my shoulders because I am scared*). The point is simply to have and to notice the body experience as it is right now, to choose what to do with it once it is felt, and then to take action based on your choice. There is much more on the dynamics of feeling, choosing, and acting to come but for now it is enough to know that, with TSY, we are not "processing" the emotional content of trauma or trying to "understand" trauma in the usual sense of the word. The suggestion is that there may be great therapeutic value in not turning what is felt in the body into a story or into an emotion. In this way, the somatic techniques I have presented all end up turning body experiences into cognitive ones where the end result involves understanding what we do with our body now in relation to the trauma we experienced in the past. With TSY, we offer our clients the opportunity to do something different, namely, instead of meaning making in our head, we are after having an experience in our body. What I invite readers to consider is whether there is room in trauma treatment for body experiences that we don't have to make meaning out of but simply notice and interact with. Our work with TSY suggests that there is and that such experiences may significantly add to the process of recovery and healing.

## Theoretical underpinnings of TSY

TSY is not based simply on the intuition that having body experiences may be helpful as part of trauma treatment. Three theoretical underpinnings to TSY-trauma theory, neuroscience, and attachment theory-come directly from the clinical literature. Let's look at each one in some detail.

### Trauma theory
Like yoga, trauma also has an ancient tradition. It has been written about and speculated upon within cultures all around the globe for millennia: from ancient epic poems, to

philosophical speculation, to treatment interventions. It has been called many things and understood in many ways but surely, since the beginning of history, humans have experienced trauma in the form of overwhelming, terrifying, and life-altering experiences. For our purposes, while it is useful to consider the fact that our forebears have been dealing with trauma forever and that it is not a new phenomenon by any means, we can skip ahead to the modern medical model that began to distinguish trauma as a treatable, psychological disorder, which occurred in the late 1970s. Specifically, we will be concerned with the following iterations of trauma: posttraumatic stress disorder (PTSD), complex posttraumatic stress disorder (CPTSD), disorders of extreme stress not otherwise specified (DESNOS), complex trauma, and developmental trauma disorder (DTD). My argument will be that all of these classifications of trauma are interrelated, build on and inform one another, and point in the direction of a similar phenomenon: trauma that occurs within the context of relationships is especially devastating to human beings and, because of its multifaceted impacts, requires a broad matrix of healing modalities.

**PTSD IS JUST THE BEGINNING**

The modern understanding of trauma starts with PTSD so let's begin there. PTSD is currently the most common terminology associated with psychological trauma because, as of the writing of this book, it is the only official diagnosis directly associated with trauma as indicated by the Diagnostic and Statistical Manual of Mental Disorders, Fifth Edition (DSM-5) or the Physicians' Desk Reference. PTSD is, therefore, the only diagnosis directly associated with psychological trauma that is presently recognized by insurance companies so it is the only trauma-related condition that can be directly billed for by clinicians. Pausing to note this monetary correlation is important, though I will not extrapolate further.

The PTSD diagnosis itself was conceived in the United States in the late 1970s and codified in the DSM-III in 1980 by clinicians who were mostly treating male combat veterans of the war in Vietnam (Andreasen, 2010). For our purposes the most notable component of PTSD is that the diagnosis is based on symptoms (e.g., recurring flashbacks, avoidance of memories associated with the events, etc.) and does not consider the specific circumstances of a survivor other than that he or she perceived a direct threat to personal safety or witnessed someone else in a life-threatening situation. In other words, whether the triggering event was a tornado, a car accident, a physical assault, or domestic violence doesn't matter from the viewpoint of the PTSD diagnosis.

After the diagnosis was established, a new door was opened for people who were suffering greatly to receive treatment, which is undoubtedly good. But the story didn't end there. Astute therapists like Lenore Terr and Judith Herman and their contemporaries noticed differences between the official diagnosis that was supported by the medical establishment and the people they actually saw in their offices. Specifically, what seemed to be missing was context. That is, a patient who had experienced a single car accident may qualify for PTSD but she had different symptoms than either patients who had been repeatedly abused within the context of relationships or survivors of repeated torture at the hands of other people. Judith Herman in particular began to call attention to trauma that occurs within the context of relationships and also has a longitudinal quality to it (there is more than one traumatic event). Herman used the word "captivity" to describe such conditions and she pointed out that people who were traumatized in captivity displayed particular symptoms, such as self-injury, explosive anger, amnesia for traumatic events, shame, preoccupation with relationship with the perpetrator, repeated failures of self-protection, and alterations in systems of meaning. Most of these symptoms that Herman saw in her experience as a psychiatrist were not described under PTSD in the DSM. In order to account for her actual experience in her office, Judith Herman needed to come up with a new framework, which she called Complex Posttraumatic Stress Disorder (CPTSD) (Herman, 1992).

**BEYOND PTSD**

The next evolution in terms of the classification of psychological trauma came because clinicians began to see a connection between complex symptoms in adulthood and traumatic experiences in childhood. The clinical observation of these consistent yet very broad symptoms led to a classification called Disorders of Extreme Stress Not Otherwise Specific (DESNOS). Again, like CPTSD, DESNOS was not an official diagnosis but rather a phenomenon that grew out of the actual experience of clinicians treating traumatized people. Eventually, there was a DESNOS symptom set developed that in some cases overlapped with that of CPTSD, but it also added some new dimensions to the literature that have bearing on the development of TSY like self-destructive behavior and chronic pain (both symptoms that play themselves out within the body) (Luxenberg, Spinazzola, & van der Kolk, 2001).

Over the next several years, DESNOS was studied, written about, expanded on, and eventually absorbed into the clinical milieu under a new name: complex trauma. Complex trauma added another important clinical observation to the mix that was referred to as "the cascading interplay between trauma exposure, impact and (mal)adaptation" (Spinazzola, Habib, et al., 2013). That is, one traumatic experience had a tendency to snowball and lead to more traumatic experiences. The cascading effect of trauma could be understood in the case of a child who was chronically physically abused at home and skipped school regularly because he didn't want anyone to see his bruises and as a result is held back a year or placed in a remedial program because he is so far behind his peers. Being in remedial programs may lead to ostracization by peers and judgment from adults, which in turn may lead to more antisocial behavior and so on. In addition to the very important concept of the cascading effect, complex trauma also arrived at a consistent and very detailed symptom array that applied to adult survivors of chronic childhood abuse and neglect, including, to name just a few, social isolation, difficulty localizing skin contact, problems knowing and describing internal states, distinct alteration in states of consciousness, substance abuse, acoustic and visual perception problems, and shame and guilt (Cook, Spinazzola, et al., 2005). These symptoms, which expand on DESNOS, add to the increasingly nuanced understanding of psychological trauma that has evolved since the late 1970s, when PTSD was first indoctrinated into medical parlance.

The final, and most current, iteration of psychological trauma that is relevant to the development of TSY is Developmental Trauma Disorder (DTD). DTD is a diagnostic framework that focuses attention on people who are exposed to trauma in the context of relationships, like CPTSD, but specifically refers to the experiences of children, like DESNOS and complex trauma. Specifically, DTD is a proposed diagnosis that would apply to children and would be entered into the DSM. The symptom array is based on the literature from DESNOS and complex trauma, and this clinical understanding would inform the treatment protocol (Ford, Grasso, et al., 2013). The symptoms, which will now sound familiar, that are cited by experts wishing to include DTD as an official diagnosis include dysregulation of affect and behavior, disturbances of attention and consciousness, distortions of self-perception, and interpersonal difficulties, along with some still inconsistent but notable changes in the brain (D'Andrea, Ford, et al., 2012). In addition, the DTD framework would presuppose the interrelational aspect of trauma because these kinds of traumas always occur within the context of relationships: specifically, adults with power and children without power.

I consider the iteration of trauma first presented by Judith Herman right up through to DTD as ultimately attempting to characterize one phenomenon, which consists of several parts where each part ends up supporting and informing the whole. Therefore, I specifically use the term complex trauma from here on out to represent this integrated phenomenon because the term seems to have, more or less, encompassed all of the other frameworks in the current clinical literature.

## EMPOWERMENT IN THE CONTEXT OF TRAUMA TREATMENT

As Judith Herman began to elucidate interrelational and longitudinal trauma as a phenomenon, she also sought to identify aspects of treatment that were particularly important. One such aspect of treatment that she identified, which is particularly relevant to TSY, she framed as follows: "No intervention that takes power away from the survivor can possibly foster recovery, no matter how much it appears to be in her immediate best interest" (Herman, 1992, p. 133). She pointedly asks us to consider power dynamics in the process of treating traumatized individuals. Power dynamics are always a relational issue but have two distinct aspects: interrelational and intrarelational. Interrelational power dynamics take place between two people: who has power in the relationship and who does not? How is power assigned in a relationship? Intrapersonal power dynamics are about my relationship to myself: how do I feel about and relate to myself? Can I change my circumstances? Can I change the way I feel if I want to? Both of these kinds of relationships are critical to the use of TSY in the treatment of complex trauma. TSY facilitators must always consider the following: is what I am doing empowering or disempowering for my client? Yoga, like therapy, can be either empowering or disempowering. I would suggest that one way for yoga to be disempowering, especially in the context of trauma treatment, is for people to be told what to do with their bodies. With TSY we are trying to create a space where our clients can experiment with doing something safe with their bodies and practice feeling what they feel without being told what to do. It is very tempting for yoga teachers to think they know what is best for their students and this is a tendency we want to shine a light on and eliminate from TSY. If we tell our clients what to do or what to feel with their bodies, even if "it appears to be in their best interest", we are not contributing to empowerment but rather reinforcing the disempowering trauma paradigm where people aren't in charge of validating their own experiences.

Empowerment, in the context of TSY, involves giving our clients the space to have their own experiences without anything being imposed from the outside-namely, your experience or your ideas about what an experience within a yoga form might or should be. As we will see later, it is important for you, the TSY facilitator, to have your own genuine experience with the forms but not to impose it on your client.

## The neuroscience of trauma

> One thing was clear: the rational, executive brain, the mind, the part that needs to be functional in order to engage in the process of psychotherapy, has very limited capacity to squelch sensations, control emotional arousal, or change fixed action patterns.
>
> —Bessel van der Kolk, 2006, p. 5

A large part of the story of the development of TSY involves current directions in neuroscience. Although the field is still in its very early stages, researchers are developing a picture of what happens to the mammalian brain as a result of exposure to traumatic experiences and it is quite devastating (Bossini, Tavanti, Calossi, et al., 2008; Long, Duan, Xie, et al., 2013). While significant impacts are being observed on many regions of the brain as a result of trauma exposure, the most important neurophysiological support for TSY is found in a set of brain regions collectively referred to in the literature as "the pathways of interoceptive awareness," or the "interoceptive pathways," which include parts of the insular cortex and the anterior cingulate cortex among others (Khalsa, Rudrauf, Feinstein, & Tranel, 2009). The term interoception will figure predominantly throughout the rest of this book and will be examined in detail in Chapter 2 but, for the moment, consider interoception as an attentional praxis that centers on our ability to feel the activity of our interior self, that is, the self contained within our skin. For example, it is interoception to feel our heartbeat, our stomach grumble, or a muscle stretch. One interesting way to understand interoception comes from the neuroscientist A. D. (Bud) Craig, who writes that it is interoceptive information that helps us develop an experience of what he calls our "sentient self" (Craig, 2010). Interoception gives us a cortical representation of our embodied self. Of particular importance to trauma treatment, researchers are finding that parts of the brain associated with our ability to interocept are deeply compromised by trauma. For example, in a script-driven, symptom-provocation study, the neuroscientist Ruth Lanius and her colleagues found that "subjects with PTSD showed lower levels of brain activation than comparison subjects in the thalamus, the medial prefrontal cortex and the anterior cingulate gyrus [parts of the interoceptive pathways]" (Lanius, Williamson, Densmore, et al., 2001, p. 1921). In another study involving combat veterans, it was found that the group with PTSD had less volume of gray matter in the left insula and the anterior cingulate than their non-PTSD counterparts (Herringa, Phillips, Insana, & Germain, 2012). This and other research are pointing to the fact that trauma survivors are deeply disconnected from their core being-the feeling of being embodied-and this seems to be a great source of the suffering associated with complex trauma and PTSD. In essence, this research on the brain suggests that traumatized people do not have a reliable self, a feel-able self, a foundation from which to safely experience themselves, relationships, and the world around them. What is it like to live in a body that is unfeel-able and therefore unpredictable? I would suggest that living with an unfeel-able and unpredictable body is one valid way to explain what complex trauma is.

Another piece of relevant neuroscience research comes from Bessel van der Kolk's lab where trauma patients were exposed to traumatic reminders and researchers found "a relative deactivation in the left anterior prefrontal cortex, specifically in Broca's area, the expressive speech center in the brain, the area necessary to communicate what one is thinking and feeling" (van der Kolk, 2006, p. 2). So, neuroscience not only presents a picture of traumatized people being alienated from their bodies but also indicates that they may be unable to talk about their experience because of the impact to Broca's area. The suggestion here is twofold: we need to pay more attention to what it really feels like to live in a traumatized body and we need a broader range of treatments for traumatized people other than those that are talk-based or strictly cognitive.

At the Trauma Center in 2011, under the direction of Bessel van der Kolk, we conducted a 20-week trial with a small group of eight adults with complex trauma. All of our subjects underwent a functional magnetic resonance imaging (fMRI) scan and then six people participated in 20 weeks of TSY. After 20 weeks, all eight participated in another fMRI scan and indications were that the group that received TSY had more activity in parts of the interoceptive pathways (left insula, right thalamus, and right dorsomedial prefrontal cortex) than their counterparts. This is an intriguing early step that we hope to investigate further.

## Attachment theory

> An infant whose mother's responsiveness helps him to achieve his ends develops confidence in his own ability to control what happens to him.                    —Mary Ainsworth, 1979, p. 933

The final theoretical underpinning of TSY comes from attachment theory, a framework that is particularly attuned to the role of relationships both in creating complex trauma in the first place and in the possibilities relationships provide in terms of healing. In a way, attachment theory developed on a parallel track to trauma theory but at some point along the way these two tracks have intersected and, in many ways, merged. Attachment theory describes a specific way of understanding the importance of relationships that has made its way directly into the treatment of complex trauma (Blaustein & Kinniburgh, 2010; Kinniburgh, Blaustein, & Spinazzola, 2005). One aspect of attachment theory that will ring a clear associative bell with complex trauma is that it seeks to understand behavior in adulthood as being directly related to the experience one has in their primary relationships in infancy and childhood. Pioneers in the field, particularly Mary Ainsworth and John Bowlby, focused mostly on the relationship between mother and child though, since their work, the understanding of "primary" relationships has expanded beyond just the biological mother (Karen, 1998). Colleagues at the Trauma Center and others who focus on attachment in the context of trauma suggest that, as helpless infants, human beings rely completely on the relationships with their primary caregivers for creating the safety that will allow them both to survive and, critically, to fully develop their capacities. Without this relational safety and stability, a human being needs to use all of his or her energy purely for survival and will therefore end up sacrificing a significant amount of normal, healthy development (Kinniburgh, Blaustein, & Spinazzola, 2005). Studies have shown that, as a result of this tradeoff-healthy development for survival-the adolescent or adult survivor will experience devastating impacts that will affect their health and well-being on many levels unless attended to effectively (see the Adverse Childhood Experiences (ACE) study data for some examples, which can be found at www.cdc.gov/ace/).

So how does TSY correspond to attachment theory? First, the trauma-informed clinical community, part of the environment from which TSY sprung, has been deeply concerned with treating the impacts of disturbed, or insecure, attachment for years (among other examples previously cited, see Courtois & Ford, 2012). Everything that happens in TSY happens within the context of a relationship-that is, the relationship between the facilitator/clinician/therapist and the student/client/patient. TSY offers many unique relational opportunities that are particularly apropos to treating attachment-based, complex trauma. First and foremost, the student is in charge of what he is doing with his body at all times so, even though the facilitator may offer some yoga-based invitations, the student can always say "yes" or "no" at any point in the process. Being in control of what you do with your body in the context of a relationship is particularly important in the treatment of complex trauma because the dysregulation associated with early childhood trauma is primarily body based. That is, when an infant or child is neglected or abused, those experiences are absorbed by the body, especially if they occur prior to the ability to verbalize (van der Kolk, 2006). For example, when the infant is hungry and the parent is repeatedly unable to supply nourishment (for whatever reason), the infant experiences an unmet body need; when the child is physically and/or sexually abused by the person she wants and needs to trust above all others to keep her safe, the body absorbs the impact of these extremely confusing messages. Pain, pleasure, terror, and a desire to please may be all mixed up and experienced within the body (consciously or unconsciously). It may be that these body feelings become so overwhelming or confusing or disorganized that eventually they become intolerable and therefore banished to the realm of the unfelt and unknown.

With TSY, we focus on using the relationship to give our clients a safe space to begin to feel their body again and begin to notice what they want to do with their body in a given situation. The facilitator supports their clients as they learn to trust what they feel, make their own choices about what to do based on what they feel, and take action based on what they choose to do. Facilitators also invite clients to notice how it feels once they take that action and then repeat the process. This is, after all, the work of a good parent or primary attachment figure: helping children notice what they feel; figure out how to act on what they feel; take action; and then help them notice how the result of their action feels. I am not suggesting that the TSY facilitator is positioning himself or herself in the role of a parent, but we should borrow from the understanding that a healthy relationship, which supports inquiry, making choices, and learning from the actions that we take, is a good paradigm to begin with when facilitating TSY.

Critically, in our experience, for most of the people we work with, this process is broken down at some stage and it is the job of any helper-including a therapist or a TSY facilitator-to assist people back into the flow, so to speak. To be out of the flow, to not know what we feel, what we want, or what to do about it is a very frightening and painful way to live. With TSY, we are always working with body sensation and dynamics and not feelings of hunger or thirst (also feelable things), for example, but researchers hypothesize that the interoceptive pathways that allow me to feel that I am hungry are more or less the same that help me feel my leg muscles contract or extend (Craig, 2003). If this is the case, then when I practice feeling my leg muscles I am toning my ability to feel/sense myself in other ways. If practitioners are aware of attachment theory, they can use the relationship to create a safe space where the client's experience is validated and supported and not coerced, manipulated, judged, or neglected.

## Try an exercise: The Seated Mountain Form

Perhaps it's best to try an exercise at this point as a way of bringing together several of the concepts that have been discussed thus far, because TSY is, ultimately, an experiential practice. If you like, we can experiment with the Seated Mountain as an example.

In order to create a form like the one pictured in Figure 1.1, the facilitator could say "sit up tall." That could be the end of it. But what would that mean in the context of trauma treatment? Perhaps the student's experience of such an instruction would be, "Well, here we go again. I am being told what to do with my body. That's familiar territory." This kind of "instruction" effectively mimics and may reinforce the trauma paradigm that was learned, maybe through the primary relationship, namely, "You are helpless to affect your circumstances, don't bother to try" or "Do what I say or else," and so on. I would suggest, based on the theoretical underpinnings presented above, that talking to one's client like this is traumatizing him or her. If we respect the impacts of complex trauma, including neuroscience, as well as the power of attachment, of the relationship, we might think differently about how we organize our presentation of the

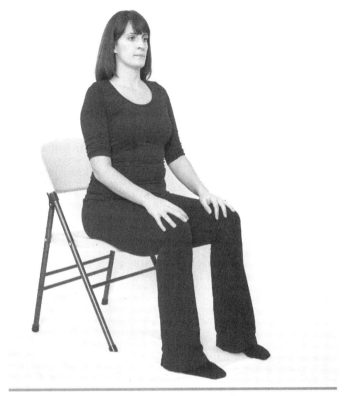

**Figure 1.1.** Seated Mountain form

Seated Mountain Form. We might notice that, through this yoga form, we have an opportunity to establish a new kind of relationship, one where the person in charge (the facilitator) turns over control to the person with less power (the client). What happens when what the client feels in the body during a yoga form is immediately validated by the therapist/facilitator? Where the client's experience is not manipulated or coerced, just validated? What happens when the client gets to make real choices about what to do with the body and is then supported in this process by the facilitator?

How might this look for our example above? The facilitator might say, "If you like, you could experiment with sitting up tall. Perhaps you might investigate lengthening up gently through the top of your head." At the same time as the facilitator is giving this invitation to the client, she is also experimenting with the same dynamics and having her own genuine experience. The process begins as an invitation, not as a command, and both parties are immediately engaged on equal footing. The facilitator might then invite her student to notice what it feels like to sit up tall: "you may feel some of the muscles that you are using to create this 'tallness' in your body." The door is immediately opened for the client to have an interoceptive experience, to feel something. Subsequently, he may or may not tell the facilitator about his experience. The important thing in the moment is that the facilitator is inviting experience, not commanding it. It would be perfectly fine, within the context of TSY, to directly ask the client some questions like "Do you feel some muscles that you are using to help yourself sit up tall?" or, even more pointedly, "Do you feel some stomach muscles engaged here?" as long as answers are not demanded, anticipated, or required. These kinds of direct questions may be helpful with some clients to, in effect, jump-start interoception but they run the risk of being coercive, so the encouragement is to proceed with caution and to always make space for the client to feel something totally different than what you are inquiring about or nothing at all without any judgment on your part.

## Bringing together trauma theory, neuroscience, and attachment theory

To wrap up this discussion of the theoretical underpinnings of TSY, I would suggest that the word that underlies trauma theory, neuroscience, and attachment theory is relationship-relationship with the other and relationship with the self. When you consider the implications of neuroscience, for example, and the impact that trauma seems to have on the pathways of interoception in particular, it is clear that, with regards to complex trauma, we are dealing with a damaged relationship to the self. Through the lens of attachment theory we recognize the impact of relationships with others both in the process of creating trauma and in the process of healing it. In this regard, I like to view Judith Herman's emphasis on empowerment in trauma healing as a bridge from neuroscience to attachment theory: how do our relationships with others impact our relationships with ourself? Do we learn to be disempowered through our dysfunctional early relationships and then re-create that dysfunction through our relationships to ourself going forward? Might this be another way to understand complex trauma? The literature around complex trauma and attachment theory suggests exactly this: it is within the context of our early relationships that we lay out a roadmap for how to relate to ourselves for a lifetime; the suffering associated with abusive or neglectful early relationships is perpetuated, ad infinitum, through the relationships with ourself. Unless we do something about it.

Nowhere is the relationship between early relational trauma and later life dysfunction more apparent than in the work of the ACE study. (To date, there have been dozens of research papers generated from the ACE data set. Interested readers can visit www.cdc.gov/ace/ to view papers.) This collaboration between the Centers for Disease Control and Prevention, and Kaiser Permanente in California clearly indicates that the more someone is exposed to chaos in childhood—violence, abuse, drugs, alcohol, neglect, and so forth—the more likely he or she will experience cognitive impairment, higher risk behaviors, heart disease, and even early death. These adverse health outcomes can be understood, when coupled with our growing knowledge of the neurophysiological impacts of trauma, as resulting from an inability for survivors to be interoceptive and to therefore be able to make informed choices about what to do with their bodies. The only way to have our needs met, whether it's medical care, nutrition, or healthy affection, is for us to be able to sense the messages from our bodies; TSY offers a starting point for that kind of interoceptive practice. With TSY we want to attend to relational dynamics-both with the other and with the self-at all times and we want to do our best to purposefully relate to our students/clients in a way that helps them build safer, more satisfying relationships to their core selves and thereby make healthier choices that result in more positive outcomes. The way we do this is by never telling our students what to do with their bodies, focusing on interoception, always using invitations instead of commands, and giving genuine options and choices within forms.

Finally, it is important to note that there are indications that while relationships can be the problem they can also be part of the solution. In a highly relevant study with foster children who showed signs of insecure attachment, foster parents were taught relational techniques like following a child's lead (very much like the TSY approach of never telling people what to do and emphasizing invitation and choice). The children who experienced these kinds of nurturing techniques from their foster parents showed lower levels of blood cortisol (a stress hormone) and improved behavioral outcomes as opposed to the control group (Dozier, Peloso, Lindhiem, et al., 2006). However, this study involved infants and toddlers while TSY is developed primarily for adolescents and adults, and it also included some age-appropriate hugging and cuddling from the caregivers (not from a third party, like a therapist or yoga teacher) and this likely had an effect on the outcomes. Still, indications are that even if insecure attachment is the first experience, humans can adapt and heal when given appropriate relational encounters later in life.

Another study examined a treatment for children and adolescents that emphasized one particular aspect of a relationship that involves the person with the most power trying to sense the emotional state of the person with less power and honoring that state rather than attempting to change it (Becker-Weidman 2006). The emphasis is again placed on the dyadic relationship, in this case between the therapist and client, and indications were that children who experienced this kind of intentional attunement from their therapist showed improvement in both affect regulation and the ability to form new social relationships. With TSY, even though our emphasis is not on the emotional state but rather on our interoceptive awareness, because the teacher is following the lead of the client, there is a type of attunement at the core of the experience (I will discuss the kind of attunement that TSY emphasizes in more detail in Chapter 6).

## Important note on the role of the facilitator

Though the role of the TSY facilitator will become more clear as you read on, I feel it is important for readers to begin to think about the practical side of using this material right at the outset. Ultimately, in order to be effective for your clients, you must have enough comfort and familiarity with the material to facilitate a coherent experience. To that end, I devote Chapter 8 to specific practices that can be used either exactly as they are presented or can be modified to suit your own experience. It will help immensely if prospective TSY facilitators practice this material themselves as well as practice teaching friends, family, and/or colleagues as often as possible. You do not have to be a yoga teacher in order to successfully use TSY as part of a therapy practice but you do need to have a practiced facility with the material. The more experience you have, the more effective you will be.

Additionally, being a facilitator for your client's body experience may be a very different role than what you are used to as a therapist so it is worth taking some time to reflect on where you are coming from. Were you trained in a very strict psychoanalytic or psychodynamic, talk-oriented approach that centers on meaning making? Are you based in a more cognitive-behavioral understanding of trauma treatment, which emphasizes the analysis of thinking and/or behavioral patterns and then an attempt to change them? Do you have some kind of somatic training? Have you ever facilitated any kind of body experience with students or clients? Are you a yoga teacher or do you have some other kind of similar training? All of these questions are important ones to consider as you contemplate how TSY might fit into your particular clinical practice.

## Shared, Authentic Experience

One critically important aspect of your role as a TSY facilitator is that you are entering into a *shared, authentic experience* with your client. That is, with any TSY exercise, the facilitator and the student are both doing the activity and it is not a situation where the facilitator is prescribing something and then standing outside of it to observe or interpret the outcome. TSY involves both parties engaging simultaneously with the material. We encountered some of the aspects of this dynamic when we discussed attachment theory. John Bowlby, the "grandfather" of attachment theory, referred to a concept that he termed mutual enjoyment as being a critical part of successful relationships. Though he referred specifically to an aspect of the mother-child relationship, I would suggest that we can broaden this understanding to consider certain aspects of any successful therapeutic relationship as well, including that between the TSY facilitator and student. In the domain of TSY, mutual enjoyment means that both parties are actively involved in the process together. So, for example, if the exercise is a Gentle Spinal Twist (see Figure 8.4 in Chapter 8), you are both doing the form at the same time. Even more important, when the facilitator invites the student to notice what he feels in his body, to practice making choices, or to experiment with taking actions (more to come on these topics in later chapters), the facilitator is also doing these things. This kind of approach adds an integrity to the practice that goes beyond words. By engaging with your client like this, you are letting her know that she is not alone, that you are both human beings with bodies that can move in some way. When you authentically model this attention to your own internal experience and do not attempt to control or coerce the experience of your client, you are letting her know that she doesn't have to "perform" for you; that she doesn't have to "get a form right" in order to please some external authority; and that she can risk being authentic in her relationship with you and her relationship with herself.

A further challenge for you is to recognize and to trust your own actual experience, as it is, without imposing it on the client. As you practice recognizing and trusting your own felt experience, you simultaneously support clients by example as they practice recognizing and trusting theirs. You share this investigation but not the outcome. You may feel one thing while they feel something else. You honor both of your experiences as equally valid. To me this coincides, a little abstrusely but none the less, with Bowlby's assertion that successful relationships contain mutual enjoyment. Complex trauma is a phenomenon of having one's experience held hostage to the whims of an external force, namely, another person. Power is largely externalized in the form of that other person. Healing trauma involves reclaiming the locus of control and, therefore, the validity of one's own felt experience. TSY is a process of internalizing power because both parties are involved in a relationship where each gets to have his or her own experience validated without imposing it on the other. To be sure, as the clinician, you are not asking for your client to validate your experience but you don't have to because you are validating it for yourself. Ultimately, your student does not need to refer to you for validation, but can instead find validation from within.

## Conclusions

To this point, I have written some about who will benefit most from TSY but it is also useful to remind readers who TSY might not be for. Though I am not a diagnostician and do not suggest that TSY be ruled out completely, this treatment was not developed for people who experienced a single-incident trauma like a car accident or a natural disaster (some exceptions might be single-incident sexual assault or any circumstance where one person purposefully hurts another). In general, single incidents are cases where techniques like eye movement desensitization and reprocessing (EMDR) may be far more effective and appropriate (Shapiro, 2001).

TSY is especially for people with complex trauma, for people who were hurt and abused continually within relationships. While our empirical data for TSY to date has focused on adult women who experienced chronic childhood abuse and neglect, we also use TSY with men with a similar background, with younger children and teens with a similar background, and with war veterans because there seem to be many similarities between these groups in terms of symptoms (see, for example, the detailed report by Davy, Dobson, et al.

[2012] on the effects of combat exposure in the Australian Defense Forces, which indicates symptoms similar to some of those found in the complex trauma literature). We are not the first to observe these similarities. Judith Herman, in her seminal book, focuses on both women trapped in abusive relationships as well as war veterans and survivors of torture. Similarly, Lenore Terr, another pioneer in the field of trauma studies, concentrated on children who experienced captivity by people other than primary caregivers (Terr, 1992). For his part, Ed Tick investigates how deeply combat experiences have affected veterans of modern war since Vietnam (Tick, 2005).

Finally, consider the image of "the yoga guru" perched on an elevated platform, in front of a room full of students, calling out directions to his rapt novitiates; students diligently follow orders as they move their bodies from one form to the next based on each successive command. This image is the antithesis of TSY because complex trauma can be similarly understood as an experience, in one way or another, of being told what to do (and what to feel) by some externalized authority, of subjugating your will to the will of another over and over again. Imagine being in these life situations: a baby born to a drug-addicted parent who is unable to meet the complex physical and emotional needs of an infant; an adult trapped in an abusive relationship; a soldier pinned down behind a wall while people try to kill him and his friends in a hail of bullets and bombs, while amid this chaos he pulls the trigger and people die. In each case, you are exposed to actions perpetrated upon, through, or withheld from your body by an external force over which you have no control. People who are steeped in chaotic environments like this learn that they are never safe in relation to other people because other people are not safe; most insidiously, as a result of these kinds of traumas, people learn that they are never safe in relation to themselves, in their own skin. Those people are who TSY is for.

Now that we have established some foundations of TSY in comparison to regular yoga and to other somatic models for trauma treatment, and investigated the theoretical underpinnings of the intervention, let's turn our attention to the methodology: how it's actually done.

# 2

# INTEROCEPTION: SENSING THE BODY

*NOTE: Chapters 2 through 7 will begin with practice examples.*

CINDY IS 39 YEARS OLD, AND SHE GREW UP IN AN AFFLUENT suburb. Her trauma history includes significant, sustained sexual and verbal abuse from her biological father, who was a very powerful, prominent public figure in town. The abuse began in very early childhood and continued into her early teens until her father committed suicide. As a child, Cindy was told over and over by her father that she or her mother would be killed if she ever told anyone about what was happening. When Cindy began to practice trauma-sensitive yoga (TSY) she had been in therapy for two decades and, although very successful in her professional life, still suffered tremendously from, among other things, an inability to sleep without intrusive nightmares, binge eating followed by prolonged periods of self-imposed starvation, cutting and burning her arms and legs, and severe dissociation that would often end up leading to major alcohol binges where she would wind up in unwanted sexual relationships with strangers. Cindy had told her therapist that she was "terrified of her body" and that she felt like her body was "only there to cause . . . pain" and many other similar things over the years. TSY was a last resort for Cindy ("I've tried everything else, why not!") and was undertaken with her therapist with whom she had a very good relationship for the prior 5 years. Cindy and her therapist decided to use TSY as a 15-minute practice at the start of each session and then they moved into the talking process that they had established over the years. During the fourth session that included TSY, Cindy and her therapist were experimenting with flexing and extending their fingers (making fists and then alternately spreading out their fingers) and noticing what that felt like. As soon as the therapist invited Cindy to notice if she felt her hands in any way, Cindy became very distressed. She said in a panic, "I can't feel anything! These hands don't seem to belong to me. There is no connection. This is really disturbing." The therapist invited Cindy to look at her hands if she wanted and to continue to experiment with moving her fingers and notice if this helped her be aware of her hands at all but Cindy said she still couldn't feel anything and was clearly still very distressed. At that point, Cindy said, in a very childlike voice, "It may be because I was tied down by my wrists so many times as part of my abuse." At this point, the therapist could have stopped the TSY altogether and shifted into another mode, possibly talking about this memory and processing it in some way. Cindy also could have called it off right there either explicitly or implicitly—she could have dissociated, for example, which would have required a shift in dynamics. But what the therapist decided to do, and what seemed acceptable to Cindy on this occasion, was to stay with TSY but shift away from the hand movements to something else. The therapist used the following language: "Would you like to experiment with a different movement?" Cindy said, "Yes, let's try the neck movements." Cindy had found over the previous few months that moving her neck had been soothing in some way and, remembering that, she initiated a shift to the neck movements in this moment of distress. So, following Cindy's lead, they began some gentle neck circles together and after a few seconds the therapist asked, "Do you feel this movement around your neck?" and Cindy said, noticeably relieved, "Yes, I can feel that." They stayed with the neck movements for a few minutes and then ended with some shoulder movements, which Cindy, again to her relief, noticed she could feel. After about 10 minutes of neck and shoulder movements they shifted into their talk therapy.

When asked later to explain her thinking during this process, the therapist said, "I was trying to give Cindy an opportunity to feel something in her body and she came up with the neck movements herself! I just felt like the most important thing at that moment was to not abandon the body if it was tolerable and for Cindy to have an opportunity to find something that was feel-able. The goal was not even to feel 'good' or to 'calm down' but just for Cindy to have an opportunity to feel something if she could tolerate that. I felt like it was more important to make available an opportunity for her to feel her body than to process a memory at that moment as long as it was okay for her."

## What is interoception?

One of the most important concepts in TSY, and one of the most important but least-known words in the English

language, is *interoception*. In 1906, the Nobel laureate
Charles Scott Sherrington introduced three terms into medical parlance: "proprioception," "exteroception," and "interoception." Of the three, perhaps proprioception, which is
basically the awareness of one's body in relation to external objects, is the most familiar. (Proprioception is why we
don't constantly walk into walls or get into car accidents.)
Exteroception refers to awareness of any stimuli coming at us
from the outside (sights, sounds, smells, etc.). Interoception
is our awareness of what is going on within the bound-
ary of our own skin; it is intra-organismic awareness. One
researcher who has devoted a good deal of his career to
studying interoception is Alan (Bud) Craig (he coined the
term "the sentient self" in this context). As a neuroscientist, Craig has developed a picture of interoception that is in
most ways too complex for our purposes but, basically, he
and others have identified nerve fibers that run from all tissues of the body to the brain. These fibers are called "afferent" because their direction is from the viscera (the body) to
the brain as opposed to efferent fibers, which run from the
central nervous system outward to the tissues of the body.
Of these afferent nerve fibers, Craig says, "Such fibers conduct information regarding all manner of physiological conditions, including mechanical, thermal, chemical, metabolic
and hormonal status of skin, muscle, joints, teeth and viscera [internal organs]" (Craig, 2003, p. 500). Importantly,
this afferent information does not have to enter conscious
awareness to be considered interoception. It is possible for
information (like a certain chemical deficiency) from a group
of muscle cells, myocytes, to reach the brain and cause a

behavioral reaction (like eating protein) without that initial information becoming conscious. With TSY, however, we are always dealing with conscious processes; therefore, for us, we are concerned with feeling dynamics within muscles, as opposed to something that is arguably not directly accessible to consciousness like an object's specific chemical content. The latter would be considered "metabolic" information and the former "mechanical," according to Craig's definition but the important thing is that both are interoception.

For another good definition of interoception, we can turn to a 2002 review written by Clare J. Fowler in the journal *Brain* about a book called *Visceral Sensory Neuroscience* by Oliver G. Cameron. Ms. Fowler writes, "As originally defined interoception encompassed just visceral sensations but now the term is used to include the physiological condition of the entire body and the ability of visceral afferent informa-tion to reach awareness and effect behavior, either directly or indirectly. The system of interoception as a whole constitutes *the material me* and relates to how we perceive feelings from our bodies that determine our mood, sense of well-being and emotions" (Fowler, 2002, p. 1505). Ms. Fowler's definition of interoception encompasses three components that we will need to deal with: the visceral experience of feeling some-thing in my body (from a muscle contracting or lengthening, to my heart beating, to my stomach grumbling); the motiva-tion to act that the visceral feeling may initiate; and the effect of our visceral experience on our mood and emotions. Again, with TSY, we focus primarily on what Ms. Fowler calls the original definition of interoception, visceral experience, but, first, let's take a look at the other two components.

After the visceral quality of interoception there is a reference to the effect of our visceral awareness on our behavior. The suggestion is that when we feel a muscle dynamic or we feel our stomach grumble we take an action in response: we stretch a muscle if it feels tight or we go and get food. Therefore, interoceptive awareness has a purpose, namely, to get us to act. While in TSY we certainly practice receiving information (see Chapter 4) from our body and then acting based on that information, however, we also practice interoception for its own sake even if that awareness does not lead to an action outcome. Our understanding of the neuroscience of complex trauma indicates that just the practice of feeling our body experience, even if we do nothing further, has specific therapeutic value for complex trauma treatment. In other words, although in upcoming chapters I will show how to connect interoception to an action outcome, our primary approach to interoception as a critical part of trauma treatment remains visceral awareness, whether or not a subsequent action is taken.

The third element of Fowler's definition of interoception involves the emotional valence of visceral experiences. Reflecting on the example of Cindy above, interoception may have some emotional content associates with it. For Cindy, noticing that she could not feel her hands was distressing while noticing that she could feel her neck was calming. In a sense, we can understand the perceived emotional content as an interpretation of the visceral experience. This gives me an opportunity to make a clear distinction regarding the methodology of TSY. While in the therapeutic process writ large there is clearly space for the exploration of emotional valence, with TSY, as a component of treatment, we stay with the visceral experience alone. In that regard, Cindy's therapist simply invited her to notice what she felt in her hands and around her neck; she did not ask Cindy to interpret what she felt in emotional terms—that interpretation came from Cindy. In TSY, our work is to strengthen the visceral, nonemotional aspect of our interoceptive capacity, not our capacity to transform body experiences into emotions.

## Evidence for the benefits of interoception from mindfulness/meditation research

At present, almost all of the evidence (aside from our small pilot study that I referenced in Chapter 1) we have for the benefits of practicing interoception on actually changing parts of the interoceptive pathways in the brain must be extrapolated from work done in the field of mindfulness or meditation by researchers like Richard Davidson (Davidson & McEwen, 2012; Lutz, McFarlin, Perlman, Salomons, & Davidson, 2013), folks associated with the Mindfulness Based Stress Reduction Program (MBSR) in Massachusetts (Davidson & Kabat-Zinn, 2003; Holzel, et al. 2011) and Sarah Lazar (Lazar, Kerr, et al. 2005). These researchers have focused their attention on contemplative practices, such as various forms of meditation that involve the use of focused attention. The interoceptive practice within TSY is also, in this way, a contemplative practice, where the object of contemplation or focused attention is the body experience (the visceral component of interoception). It is possible to extrapolate from the findings of the meditation research that it is the practice of attentional control, regardless of whether the object of one's attention is a thought, an emotion, a sound, or a body feeling, that may have an effect on the workings of neurons and therefore brain regions associated with trauma. While this is a speculative stretch at this point, it is by no means a radical one and would surely be an area ripe for further research. Why, you may ask, if meditation has shown such promising results, do we need TSY as another option for traumatized people? Because, ultimately, meditation is a cognitive process and TSY is an interoceptive one. With meditation the body is held in a rather passive state and most of the work is done with the mind: either observing thoughts and emotions or intentionally creating certain cerebral or emotional states. In order to do meditation one must have a robust-enough frontal lobe (the executive part of the brain) in the first place to know that thoughts and feelings are just thoughts and feelings and that they will come and go or they can be changed at will. For our complexly traumatized clients, thoughts and feelings are experienced as trauma all over again and not as phenomena that can be observed without emotional and visceral reactivity (van der Kolk, 2006). Meditation, like any other kind of cognitive treatment that doesn't take self-regulation into account, is actually retraumatizing for complexly traumatized clients (for more, see the section below about interoception and self-regulation). In contrast to meditation, with TSY, the body, not the mind, is the center of activity. The conceptualization of trauma that undergirds TSY considers the problem to be more an experience of what is happening right now in the body—what it feels like to exist in this body right now—and less about thoughts about trauma or thoughts about the past or the future. Ultimately, this treatment attempts to go directly to where trauma lives: in the body.

## Practicing interoception using TSY

Now that we have an understanding of what interoception is and the framework for why we should bring it into treatment for complex trauma, let's turn our attention to ways in which we can use TSY and actually practice the sense of interoception.

### Language of interoception

In order to bring interoception into the therapeutic milieu, the facilitator has one very important tool: language. The most important interoceptive word is *notice*, as in *if you like, you can tilt your head to one side and when you do this you may notice a feeling in the side of your neck* or *if you like, notice how it feels in your lower back when you fold forward.* The general encouragement is to use the word *notice* as often as possible as long as it is tolerable to your clients. What is it that you are inviting your clients to notice? Anything that is feel-able in their body. Because it is possible to notice all kinds of things like thoughts and emotions, for example, and our focus is always on the felt experience in the body, it is important that we look a little closer at how we use language to make interoception available.

Consider again the invitation *if you like, you can tilt your head to one side and when you do this you may notice a feeling in the side of your neck.* Figure 2.1 depicts this action.

For the purpose of this chapter, let's focus on the interoceptive language (I've already talked about invitatory language in Chapter 1): *you may notice a feeling in the side of
your neck*. While *notice* is the key interoceptive word it is
not able to stand alone—we can't just randomly tell (or even
invite) our clients to "notice without suggesting something
to notice." There has to be an object of awareness and, most
of the time, we need to make that object very clear. In our
example the object is *the side of your neck*. Now your client
has something to hold onto—somewhere to direct attention.
(In the larger picture of TSY, we also want to make it clear
to our clients that they may not feel anything and that that's
perfectly ok. We are not requiring that they feel anything; we
are just making the possibility of feeling something available
to them.) So, now that we have established an object (the side
of your neck) and an initial impetus to interoception (notice),
we are still missing something. Imagine if the sentence was
*you may notice the side of your neck*. While it works as a sentence, that is, it has a subject (you), a verb (notice), and a
noun (neck), it seems incomplete for our purposes, doesn't
it? Notice *what* about the side of my neck? I have nothing
specific to notice yet (or maybe I have too much and I get
overwhelmed). In our use, the word *notice* is a verb but if it
stands alone in this sentence it is very weak, especially if we
are trying to practice interoception. We need to strengthen
this sentence so that our clients know what it is we are inviting them to notice: hence the additional words *a feeling*. Now,
*notice* is still the verb but *a feeling* becomes the subject and *in
the side of your neck* stands as the object.

You may notice a feeling in the muscles at the top of your
   legs.
You may notice a feeling in your hand.
You may notice a feeling in your lower back.

The encouragement is to use some iteration of *notice a feel-ing* as often as possible in a TSY session because this is how

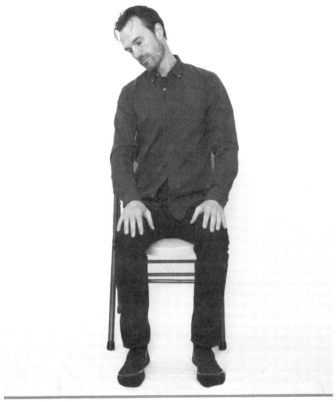

**Head Tilt**

you can most directly bring up the practice of interoception. Also the word *notice* is not replaceable in our sentences above, but the word *feeling* is. You could, for example, invite people to *notice a sensation in the side of your neck* and this would still be interoceptive practice. One final caution when it comes to language and TSY is to avoid the use of adjectives and adverbs. These two sentences are examples:

> You may notice a good feeling in the side of your neck.
> You may notice that the side of your neck feels good when you tilt to one side.

In both cases, by using a feeling word ("good") in the context of TSY, we end up coercing our clients into having a certain kind of experience (or putting our client in a position where she may feel something that she does not experience as good and is therefore in conflict, which can also damage the relationship); such coercion is antithetical to trauma treatment. Additionally, our work is to make interoception available to our clients and interoception has nothing to do with adverbs or adjectives. If your client wishes to interpret a feeling in his body as good or bad, that is fine but it is not the point of TSY, nor is it part of the role of the facilitator for reasons that I hope are becoming more clear to readers.

## No coercion

As we begin to introduce TSY into the therapeutic process it is very important that we remain conscious of one pitfall that is lurking around the edges of each yoga form: the impulse to influence your client's experience in a coercive or manipulative way. I brought up this issue in Chapter 1, and again above, but I would like to expand on it here. I call it an *impulse* because we want to help the people we are serving, we want them to get better, and any new tool, like TSY, that purports to help traumatized people get better can cause us to be a little overzealous. The key is that in order for TSY to work the facilitator must absolutely never, under any circumstances, coerce their client into doing some yoga form or another or into having a particular experience with a yoga form that the facilitator thinks will be beneficial in some way. It is very tempting as a facilitator to place external value on a form like, *this form will help you relax* or *this form will help you feel happier* or *this form will help you to feel strong.* What happens if your client doesn't feel relaxed or happy or strong in the given form? What happens to the role of interoception? There is a shift away from the internal experience and toward an external one where someone else's value of the yoga form begins to dominate. Under these circumstances it becomes unclear what our focus is in practicing TSY and in a worst-case scenario the client's actual experience with interoception is totally neglected. What the client feels in his body is devalued in favor of the expectations placed on him by the facilitator. Consider, for example, what this does to the power dynamics in the relationship. In effect, the teacher is short-circuiting the interoceptive process of the student by stepping in and saying, implicitly or explicitly, *just feel what I want you to feel* or, further, *what you actually feel is not as valid as what I suggest that you feel.* This sounds rather extreme but, I would argue, is not far off from what happens in many yoga classes that are taking place every day in health clubs, yoga studios, and ashrams around the world. Also, critically, this sounds a lot like a trauma paradigm, doesn't it? When we bring yoga into the domain of trauma treatment we must not tell people what to do or what to feel. Essentially, we are careful not to make *feeling something particular* the goal of TSY. Actually it is very important that we don't make feeling anything the ultimate goal of TSY because it is in the nature of complex trauma that there will be many times when our clients will not be able to feel certain parts of their bodies. That is totally and completely ok. In fact, please remind your client (and yourself) from time to time, "You may not feel anything in this form and that's ok." We want to make interoception explicitly available, help people discover it where they can, but we don't want to present interoception like it's required and we don't want our clients to feel in any way like they have failed if they don't feel something.

## Focus on the internal experience

To be traumatized is to live in a body with which you have an unreliable and unpredictable relationship. Where does that unreliability and unpredictability come from? In large part from our inability to interocept. As discussed in Chapter 1, we know that parts of the brain, collectively referred to as the pathways of interoception, are affected by trauma. This means that we know our traumatized clients have particular difficulty feeling their internal states and this fundamental disconnection contributes in large part to the suffering associated with trauma. If you practice TSY with your traumatized clients you present them with an opportunity to feel and sense themselves. Without a somatic intervention like this, all you can do is talk about what it is like to feel estranged from your body; you talk about someone's very real and immediate experience as an abstract cognition. These kinds of conversations may be useful at times but they are no substitute for interacting in some way with the body that is the cause of such consternation and the seat of the actual experiences! TSY gives you and your client a way to have these kinds of interactions based on the actual experience of feeling something. This is exactly what happened in our practice example with Cindy. Her therapist, sensing the benefit of staying with the body, if tolerable, so that Cindy could have a direct, feel-able experience, decided not to shut down TSY and move into a more abstract, cognitive process. Instead, Cindy's therapist kept the focus on the internal experience as it was in the moment. By staying with the internal experience, Cindy was able to discover that parts of her body were indeed feel-able and that everything that occurred within her own skin wasn't mysterious or painful.

As we introduce TSY to our clients, we seek to give them access to their bodies, knowing that their bodies are often the most frightening place of all for them. The work is to experiment with different yoga forms, as long as it is tolerable for the client, until a part of the body is revealed as accessible and feel-able.

One extra challenge in practicing interoception is that so many traumatic memories seem to be stored in the body, just outside of conscious awareness, and your clients have probably developed a keen physical infrastructure around protecting themselves from these implicit memories (Rothschild, 2000; van der Kolk, 1994, 2006). When you invite them to feel their bodies, it may be a very dysregulating experience even if it may be an essential part of trauma treatment to eventually be safe sensing your body. By using TSY to invite the body into the therapeutic milieu you will be exposing your clients to some very painful terrain, perhaps the thing they are trying most determinedly to avoid: awareness of the body. Because of these challenges, it is useful to approach interoception as a dosage issue: that is, how much interoceptive practice can my client tolerate? How much is too much? When is interoception appropriate and when is it better to talk or to use some other kind of intervention?

## Interoception and self-regulation

Self-regulation is fine as long as it does not interfere with interoception. What does this mean? Self-regulation is, simply put, our ability to calm ourselves down when we are agitated. Survivors of traumatic experiences, especially complex trauma, very often have difficulty regulating emotional and behavioral arousal (Kinniburgh, Blaustein, & Spinazzola, 2005). Therefore, many therapists believe that it is essential to help clients find ways to self-regulate. There are three big problems with self-regulation in terms of TSY methodology.

First, in most clinical contexts, self-regulation involves emotions and not visceral feelings in the body. With TSY, we are not facilitating emotional experiences; while we do not want to avoid them if they come up, we, as TSY facilitators, do not want to bring them up ourselves. Consider our case example. Cindy's therapist does not invite her to stop moving her hands because it is emotionally distressing but primarily because she couldn't feel anything; it was an interoceptive dead end. Their work was to find a part of the body that Cindy could feel.

Second, a belief like "my client needs to learn to calm themselves down when they get upset" can easily lead to a prescription like "my client needs to learn how to use his breath to self-regulate" or "my client will feel more calm if they do a forward fold." This is another trap. We always want to avoid the urge to prescribe when using TSY. TSY may offer some opportunities to practice self-regulation *but it is not the most important part of the practice nor is it even necessary.* Another way to say this is that self-regulation is fine as long as it is not prescribed. As TSY facilitators, our commitment to not telling people what to do or feel trumps our ideas about self-regulation. If your client notices that something she does helps her feel more calm, like taking a deep breath or moving into a certain yoga form (like Cindy in our example with the neck movements), that is fine and it is certainly reasonable for you, the facilitator, to reflect back to your client how great it is that she found something that helped her feel more calm. But our work is not about making ourselves feel calmer: it is first and foremost about learning to feel our bodies and the things that our bodies can do. If you as the clinician feel that the most important thing for your client right now is that he calm down, you will use a technique other than TSY (i.e., there is literature available on using breath and posture to change cortisol and testosterone levels in the body in order to calm down and feel more competent). In terms of TSY, however, feeling calm is perfectly acceptable as long as it does not trump interoception; to put it another way, feeling calm is fine as long as it comes from interoception and is not a prescription.

The third big problem with self-regulation is that if we get too side-tracked by emotions the process can quickly veer off into cognitive territory where we become hung up on interpreting body experiences through an emotional/cognitive framework: this is not TSY. While we recognize that emotional interpretation of interoceptive experiences will happen from time to time, we do not want to encourage it.

My suggestion is that if you use TSY you will create an environment where the emphasis is on interoception and where your client is in charge of his body (more on this in the next two chapters) and he will discover self-regulation techniques for himself. Critically, all of what he discovers will belong to him and will be embodied by him for the very fact that it was not prescribed. It will not be something external to be doled out like medication according to the benevolence of some "expert." Your client becomes the expert. The truth is, there will be plenty of room in therapy for talking about emotions; there will probably also be plenty of room in treatment for prescribing self-regulation techniques. You are bringing TSY in as a way to do something new, which is to practice the visceral aspect of interoception, that is, to have unmitigated, uninterpreted body experiences.

## 3

# BRINGING CHOICE
# INTO THERAPY

RANDALL IS A 16-YEAR-OLD WITH A SIGNIFICANT HISTORY
of physical abuse and neglect from his family of origin. He
was introduced to TSY as part of his weekly therapy session
in the residential treatment program where he had been living for the past year. Randall and his therapist had cocreated
a 10-minute TSY program that they would do together, usually at the beginning of a clinical session. After a period of
trial and error that lasted about 2 months, Randall had dis-
covered a set of chair-based yoga forms that he wanted to use
as a regular routine. For Randall, TSY had a lot to do with
the physical shapes of the forms and he noticed that some
body positions caused him too much pain—both physical
discomfort but also psychological and emotional discomfort.
Aware of the fact that TSY is focused on the visceral experience and not on translating body experiences into psychological or emotional content, Randall's therapist worked
mostly with helping him notice how his body felt in different
forms and then, if he was uncomfortable in any way, practicing either modifying the form so that it was more physically
comfortable or coming out of the form entirely. On this occasion, they were doing a gentle backbend together in their

chairs that involved lifting the chin toward the ceiling and rolling back the shoulders (see Figure 3.1 for a picture of this form).

Randall had previously experienced this form as one of his favorites. He had enjoyed the feeling of lifting his chin and feeling the muscles in the front of his neck stretch. On this particular occasion, as they were doing the form together, the therapist invited Randall, as he often did, to notice what he was feeling in his body by saying, "You may notice some feeling in the muscles or the space around the front of your neck." On this day, as soon as the words were uttered, Randall began to panic. "Ow!" he said. "The front of my neck really hurts." This hadn't happened to him before and it was new and unexpected. The therapist was also a bit surprised but before he could even respond to Randall's distress, Randall himself actually verbalized, "I am going to come out of this form." Fantastic! He had apparently internalized the process of choosing to come out of a form that was distressing and he could access this choice without the therapist cueing it. Normally, the therapist would have had to talk Randall through the choice process so this was also a new experience for the therapist. Randall proceeded to come out of the form but he didn't stop there. Next he said, "I know what I can do," and he folded forward with his forearms on the top of his legs, rounded his back slightly, and tucked his chin a little bit (see the form called Forward Fold, Version 1, in Chapter 8 for an example). This was another form that they had practiced together for several months. The therapist was just trying to follow Randall's lead now so he too came out of the form and gently folded forward. "How does your neck feel in this form?" the therapist asked. "Much better," Randall said, taking a deep breath. "I felt like a sharp pain in my throat in the other one but when I lean forward it totally goes away." Randall was noticeably relieved. He had internalized the capacity to make choices about what to do with his body and he noticed that not only could he stop doing something that was painful but he could also move himself into another form that felt better.

## Choice in TSY

What does it mean to make a choice? How is it that we choose one thing over another? The answers to these questions depend largely on who you ask. A neuroscientist may have one answer, a psychologist another, a philosopher yet another, and so on. In other words, each of these professional disciplines would emphasize a certain mechanism for choice making based on the area of expertise or professional bias (the function of neurons in the brain, past experience and learning, rational or irrational thinking, etc.). Readers will surely discern my own biases regarding choice making after reading this chapter. In fact, I will attempt to make some of them as clear as possible throughout the course of the book.

Along with bias, another important factor to consider regarding how we approach the process of making choices is the context, that is, are we choosing a new career path or are we choosing how high to lift our arms in a yoga form? The former is a choice that, to a large degree, involves our ideas so is therefore more cognitive (What job will best serve my financial needs? Where do I see myself professionally in 5

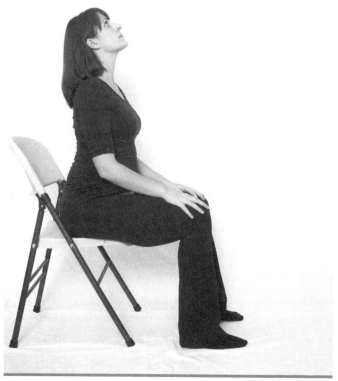

**Figure 3.1.** Gentle backbend: Lifting your chin and rolling your shoulders back.

years? What job will make me happiest after I take it?), and the latter is a choice that mostly involves our experience of how our body feels right now so it is therefore less cognitive and more visceral. As we consider the practice of making choices with regards to TSY, it is useful to distinguish between choices that are more weighted toward reasoning and those related more to immediate, somatic experience.

Additionally, these two examples—deciding on a job versus deciding how high to lift your arms in a yoga form—also illuminate another component of the choices we make, namely a temporal one. If we are thinking about a career path, we would probably be more concerned with the future (What choice will lead to my long-term happiness?) whereas how high to lift our arms in a yoga form invites more of a focus on the present (What do I want to do with my body right now?). When considering choice making and TSY, the context is our immediate body experience and the time frame is the present moment. In other words, all of the choices that we practice making in TSY are related to what to do with our body right now.

## Trauma as an extreme lack of choice

Additionally, our approach to choice making in TSY has evolved from our understanding that the kind of trauma our clients have experienced involves what can be referred to as *an extreme lack of choice*. For example, an infant born into a violent or neglectful home has no choice about those circumstances; this infant is trapped in every sense of the word. An infant born into this kind of chaotic environment would be incapable of making a conscious choice to leave such an environment (or to change it) so the lack of choice I am pointing to is even more complex and insidious than we might think at first. Consider this infant as an organism who, at this developmental stage, has mostly biological needs: nutrition, sleep, hygiene, but also, according to work related to attachment theory as we saw in Chapter 1, physical contact and the attunement of an adult caregiver. When an infant does not receive this care, attention, and affection, he or she fails to develop successfully (Ainsworth, 1979; Feldman, Eidelmann, Sirota, & Weller, 2002) and is at great risk for suffering from the effects of complex trauma years later (Anda et al., 2009). The infant is, in many ways, trapped and helpless. Perhaps we can agree that no organism would choose these conditions. No organism would subject itself willingly to an environment where it would fail to thrive and put its long-term health at risk (Corso, Edwards, Fang, & Mercy, 2008). Under these conditions it is as if the biological organism were making a desperate plea for mercy through its failure to develop in a healthy way, a plea that goes eternally unheeded because it cannot be uttered to anyone ever (there is no language) and the people most capable of understanding this language-less utterance and saving the defenseless infant are the ones who are causing all of the pain and suffering in the first place. Therefore, because the infant, the organism, is subjected to this kind of traumatizing environment without the ability to change it we can understand it as an *extreme lack of choice* and it is under these conditions that complex trauma flourishes. With TSY we counter this experience of extreme lack of choice with as many opportunities as possible for our clients to practice making real choices about what to do with their bodies.

## Is it adaptation or choice?

Complex trauma has been described as a "cascading interplay between trauma exposure, impact and (mal)adaptation" (Spinazzola, et al., 2013, p. 8). As discussed in Chapter

1, trauma does not end with the event itself or the events themselves. Rather, particularly with complex trauma, the event is just the beginning because it will reverberate throughout our lives (the impact) and we do our best to adapt (or maladapt as it were). For example, research has shown that people who experience childhood trauma are at increased risk for dangerous behaviors such as drug taking (Dube, et al., 2003; Khoury, et al., 2010) and self-harm (Yates, 2004). While these dangerous behaviors can be understood as adaptations to the early traumatic experience, it is also true that society often has another interpretation that it operates from, which is important for us to consider. I contend that society in general most often looks on these *adaptations* to trauma as more of a product of free will. To an outside, uninformed observer, it appears as if we choose to take drugs, to cut ourselves, to engage in dangerous sexual relationships, and so on, as if we see a wide array of options for ourselves and are willfully picking. This isn't the most honest way to understand what's happening. It is my position that our traumatic experiences, being aberrations themselves, perform an insidious sleight of hand and effectively replace our free choices with adaptive responses. To the external observer there is no difference but to those who understand trauma the difference is everything and is in many ways the crux of the whole problem. If we are stuck constantly adapting to trauma, and the systems around us (society) are treating us like people making free choices from a completely open slate of options, then we have the recipe for pathologizing the traumatized person instead of the trauma itself. I realize this line of argument is veering in a political direction so I will stop here but the central point is very important for the development of TSY, namely that we want to differentiate between adaptive responses and making real choices, and we want to practice the latter.

Finally, even if, in the end, we still believe that traumatized people are making choices instead of adapting to trauma I would still argue that their choices become distorted and very limited by trauma, and we can use TSY to introduce a new and safer array of choices to people.

## How to use TSY to bring real choices into therapy

There are three specific things we can do with TSY that will bring real choices into therapy:

1. Make everything an invitation instead of a command.
2. Connect choices explicitly to what can be done with the body right now.
3. Connect choices to interoception.

### Invitatory language: The language of empowerment

I mentioned the use of invitations earlier in the book but now I want to shine a light on it. How we use language with these yoga exercises makes a huge difference in how therapeutic they are in the context of trauma treatment. As a reminder, Judith Herman says, "No intervention that takes power away from the survivor can possibly foster her recovery, no matter how much it appears to be in her immediate best interest (Herman, 1992, p. 133).." The flip side of this argument is that the things we do that empower our clients foster their recovery. In the context of TSY, making every cue an invitation rather than a command is empowering. Invitations are empowering because they give people an opportunity to orient their frame of reference to their own internal experience as opposed to commands, which orient people to something external, namely the will and desire of the person in power. Consider these two statements:

1. Lift your right arm.
2. If you like, lift your right arm.

Notice what each of these statements feels like. Perhaps say them out loud to yourself. Please ask yourself the following when you consider each statement: Who is in charge? What if I don't want to lift my right arm? What kind of relational dynamics does this statement foster? The first example is a command and with a command, only one person is in charge and it is the person giving the command. Not only that, but commands foster an externalization of experience because those who receive commands are always oriented to the person in power. And, yes, commands delineate a clear power dynamic. With a command it is implied that you really don't have a choice, and we have already identified trauma itself as an extreme lack of choice. Commands reinforce the extreme lack of choice that accompanied trauma in the first place.

The second example, "if you like, lift your right arm," is an invitation and it totally shifts the locus of control from the external to the internal. The addition of the simple phrase "if you like" presents the possibility for a genuine choice to be made by the invitee. Now, each person gets to make a choice for himself or herself. There is no external authority to either please or thwart. Perhaps more subtly, invitations also remove a moralistic component from the equation because what we do becomes a choice that is relativistic whereas a command implies right and wrong: in the sense that what the commander wants you to do is "right" and anything else is "wrong." Notice how insidious this is— with a command like "lift your right arm" the *right thing* to do is to follow the order of the external authority. To not lift your right arm is to do the *wrong thing* as well as to displease the person in power. If you have a real choice then you get to refer to your own experience and what is right becomes what is right for you, not for someone else. You get to practice making a choice unabated and uninfluenced by the will of some external authority. Complex trauma is about your will being constantly subjected to an external authority. You do not get to refer to your own expertise when you are traumatized (expertise, in this case, being the answer to the question of what do *I* want?). In fact, if you are repeatedly abused or neglected it is probably better to cut yourself off from your own expertise because you don't get to use it anyway and you might as well save your energy for something more important, like survival. But what happens if we learn to live entirely disconnected from our own expertise, our own sense of what it is that we want?

With TSY we are interested in helping people refer to their own internal authority, particularly regarding what to do with their bodies, and a key way we do this is by using language to offer real invitations. We refer to this kind of language (like statement 2 above) as *invitatory language.* Our goal, and the encouragement for any clinician interested in bringing TSY into treatment, is that every cue be preceded by an invitatory phrase. Everything in TSY is an invitation and not a command and the more we can be committed to this premise the more effective the intervention will be in terms of trauma treatment. Other examples of invitatory language are "when you are ready," "you may wish to," "perhaps" (as in "perhaps, folding forward"), and "maybe" (as in "maybe taking two or three breaths in this form"). Please feel free to either use these phrases or to come up with your own that you are comfortable using as often as possible.

## Choice making as an immediate body experience

In TSY, every choice that we make is related to something that we do with our body right in the immediate moment; we are not reflecting on past choices or anticipating future decisions. We are interested only in the choices we make right now in relation to whatever yoga form we are currently engaged in. The fact that our choices are body-oriented presents a particular challenge when working with traumatized people, and this needs to be explicitly addressed and reckoned with: for most of our clients, making choices about what to do with their bodies will be very difficult due to the very nature of complex trauma itself. Most of our clients hate their bodies and/or feel extremely detached from them. We have seen some of the clinical sequelae that are probably related to this hatred or disconnection, such as changes in the brain that make it difficult to sense or to interpret body experience. We can also imagine that an abuser is demonstrating so much hate and violence toward the body of a victim that if someone is steeped in this kind of environment he or she will eventually internalize that hatred. We are after all social animals, exquisitely attuned to the lessons we learn from each other (not to mention some of the more recent research into epigenetics that seems to suggest we may inherit genes that are also, in effect, attuned to and manipulated by traumatic experiences).

Because of this a priori challenge, the general encouragement when introducing body-based choice is to start with a simple framework that we can call an "A-B choice." For example, if you would like to try an A-B choice, you are welcome to experiment with another neck exercise called head circles. With the head circles you are welcome to either do A (a half head circle) or B (a full head circle). Option A would be dropping your chin gently forward and then rolling your head from side to side. It's like the bottom half of a circle. Option B would be to make a full head circle. Feel free to pause and experiment with these movements for a moment. As you can see, these options can be presented as an A-B choice with no other objective other than choosing between A and B. For some of our clients, experimenting with these A-B choices may be enough; this alone may add a new dimension to choice making and to trauma treatment. Your client may be clearly aware of the choice she is making or she may just pick A or B seemingly at random; it doesn't matter. The encouragement is to keep offering these A-B choices as often as possible so your client gets to have the experience of making a choice in the context of her body.

Some of your clients may be interested in other aspects

of choice making, in which case you can add some complexity. For example, from the head circle exercise initiated above, the next step might involve adding more choices, as in an A-B-C model: you can do A (a half circle), B (a full circle), or C (a U-shape or horseshoe-shape movement, like a three-quarter circle). Now you have added a third option and therefore more complexity into the mix. Now your client has an opportunity to broaden her choice-making spectrum and all of it is connected to what she is doing with her body. Every yoga form presented in this book provides opportunities to practice by making various A-B and A-B-C choices.

*PRACTICE TIP: While it is possible to add even more choices to a yoga form, be careful of getting bogged down in one form for too long. If your client is starting to make it more of a cognitive exercise rather than a visceral/somatic one, take that as a signal that it is probably a good time to move on.*

## Connecting choices to interoception

Another possibility, if your client is tolerating the A-B or the A-B-C choices and seems interested in even more complex choice making, is to invite him to start to notice what he is feeling in his body and to possibly connect what he is feeling to the choices he is making. For example, given our neck role exercise, the facilitator could say, "If you like, notice what the different options feel like around your neck and maybe let that help you make your choice." This kind of invitation invites interoception into the process. Now your client has an opportunity to make a choice based on what he feels in his body. The choice process becomes anything but arbitrary. Now it is what do I feel and what do I want to do with my body based on what I feel? Figure 3.2 outlines how someone might use an A-B-C choice model combined with interoception.

**Figure 3.2.** Connecting an A-B-C choice with interoception.

Try **A** and notice how it feels. If it feels tolerable, stay with it.
If **A** doesn't feel tolerable, try **B** and notice how it feels.
If **B** feels tolerable, stay with it.
If **B** doesn't feel tolerable, try **C** and notice how it feels.

When we start to get into an interoceptive practice like this, we, as facilitators, have to be really careful to let our clients determine what does and does not feel tolerable. In fact, I use the word *tolerable* just to illustrate the point but the recommendation in practice is to just invite your client to "notice what this variation feels like" and to remind him or her that "there are also other options for this form." In other words, avoid using adjectives and adverbs like "tolerable" (or "good" or "bad," etc.) when you are actually facilitating TSY and just let your clients have their own experience. They may tell you, "This form is uncomfortable," in which case you can offer variations and invite them to notice how the variations feel. A very common experience is that a client will tell you that a form is uncomfortable but will not ask you for help. I usually experience this scenario as an effect of complex trauma where my client is used to being uncomfortable in his body and truly doesn't believe there is any other possibility available or he doesn't trust me (the authority figure) to be able or willing to help him relieve his pain. When this happens I still try to let him know there is another variation or two available for the form and I will demonstrate it myself and also remind him that he can always come out of any form for any reason. I try to meet that impact of trauma that my client is experiencing with something new: choices that can be made, which I support but do not command. Readers may be reminded of an earlier discussion from Chapter 2, where I made it a priority to not adopt a prescriptive stance toward your client where you are telling him or her what to do or feel. When you present choices like this, even though you are giving clients some possibilities, the process is still entirely nonprescriptive because you are inviting clients to notice what they feel and to be led exclusively by that experience.

**IMPORTANT NOTE:** *Please remember that even though I present choices in a way where complexity can build, any of these choice-making practices will contribute to the work of trauma healing. The role of the facilitator is not to prescribe one choice model over the other but to be led by what is tolerable or helpful for each client at a particular time. In that way you maintain the integrity of the entire process, which is for the client to learn through practice to be guided by his or her own internal experience rather than by any external influence.*

## What not to do: How physical touch foils the power of choice in TSY

Because so many yoga classes involve physical assists (that is, yoga teachers putting their hands on their students and physically manipulating their bodies) I want to make this clear statement: in TSY, there are *no* physical assists. The facilitator will never place his or her hands on a client in the context of TSY.

I would like to share two pieces of supportive evidence in this regard. The first one is anecdotal. In the early years of the yoga program at the Trauma Center, we did do physical assists. We thought it would be a good idea for trauma survivors to be able to experience "safe touch" and we didn't want people to feel "untouchable." We thought we were doing the right thing. However, we started to get some troubling feedback. Several students, both long-term folks and newcomers, told us that when we said words like "if you like" and "when you are ready," they took those words seriously. When we said, "You have a choice about how you do this form; there are options," they trusted us. They told us that as soon as we put our hands on them (even in a very gentle way) all of these nice words went out the window. The experience was "I'm doing something wrong," "the teacher is angry at me," "I need to do it your way even though my body is trying to tell me something else," or "I am now scared of you because you want me to do something with my body that I don't understand or that I don't want to do."

As soon as we heard a few of these comments, we knew we had to drop physical assists entirely when working with victims of complex trauma. What appeared to be happening was that a physical touch was sending a different message than our words, no matter how well intentioned we were. In the context of TSY, people interpreted touch as threatening and dangerous, which, looking back, is completely

understandable, given what we now know and have discussed in Chapter 1 about the impact of complex trauma
(incidentally, when we first started the yoga program at the
Trauma Center, there was no book like this to refer to so I
am hoping to save you and your clients from some of the
mistakes we made along the way). We were not honoring
choices and invitations. TSY is supposed to be a place where
you are totally, completely, unequivocally in charge of what
you do with and feel within your body and when we as the
facilitator put our hands on people we were sending the message that what our students were doing or feeling was some-
how wrong.

We as a team quickly came to believe that this experience
was sabotaging the entire process and was (at best) causing
our clients to not trust us and to either stop attending sessions or dissociate more or (at worst) retraumatizing people.
Imagine how painful it is for a trauma survivor to hear you
say "you have choices" and then to experience you physically manipulating his body just as he is making the first
tentative (and profoundly inspiring) steps to feel and make
choices about what to do with his body. Our clients are people who have survived deeply abusive and neglectful relationships and the fact that external stimuli (our touch) are
being interpreted as threatening is exactly the result that one
would expect (Blaustein & Kinniburgh, 2010), regardless
of the "good" intentions behind them. So we changed our
methodology and eliminated physical touch.

The next important piece of information that came along
later, which supported our no-touch approach, arose from
the qualitative interviews done as part of our National

Institutes of Health (NIH) study. It is very common for adult clients to tell us that being touched by their children or intimate partners is one of the worst experiences in their lives exactly because they expect it to be enjoyable; they want to enjoy hugging and cuddling their loved ones but they can't. Many of the women in our study told us that after 10 weeks of TSY (that involved no touch) they were in fact able to be touched by their children and partners whereas before TSY that touch had been unbearable (West, 2011). This is critical information. Our speculation is that by practicing real choice in an invitation-based context where you are totally in charge of your body, what you do with it, how you move it, when you move it, you begin to learn to feel safe in your own skin. Once you feel safe in your own skin, you can accept the contact of others' skin (your baby, your lover) and maybe even enjoy it. When the yoga teacher touches you in this context it sends messages of danger that override the work of choice, invitation, and interoception that actually need to be done in order for people to be able to enjoy being touched by appropriate people in their lives.

## Conclusions

In TSY, choices are something that we practice intentionally in the present moment and that are not related to thoughts about the past or the future. Choices are always connected to forms—what we are doing with our body—though they may or may not be connected to interoception. We use yoga forms as opportunities to have different physical experiences where one can make a variety of choices about what to do with the body. Our work is to do our best to create an environment where our clients are empowered to practice choice without external coercion or influence of any kind.

Now that we have established the primacy of choice in the TSY framework, we can turn our attention to the next critical practice: action.

# 4

# TAKING
# EFFECTIVE ACTION

SAM IS A 30-YEAR-OLD MALE WITH A CHILDHOOD TRAUMA history; he also was a veteran of the wars in Iraq and Afghanistan. He had been in therapy for 2 years by the time we met. At the time of this example, we had done yoga together for about 9 months. One day we were doing the Seated Mountain Form (see Chapter 8 for an example) together, and after a few minutes of sitting, Sam said, "My back feels really sore." I responded, "Would you like to try standing up?" After a moment, Sam replied, "Yeah, ok." We stood up together and I asked, "How does your back feel now?" Sam's face changed from a grimace to a smile and he said, "Hey, it feels a lot better." I then asked Sam if he wanted to try that action again and this time we could each experiment with noticing the muscles we felt that helped us move from sitting to standing. He was up for it. He was curious. So we sat back down and took a couple of breaths and then tried it again. My invitation was "if you like, moving a little more slowly this time, experiment with noticing whatever muscles you feel." Once we stood up I asked Sam if he noticed any muscles and he said, pointing to the top of his legs, "I felt these big muscles in my legs just when I started standing." I shared that I had noticed the muscles in the backs of my arms because I had pushed myself off of the arms of the chair to get started. Finally, I asked Sam again while we were still standing, "How does your back feel?" "Good, good," he said.

## From feeling and choosing to acting

In Chapters 2 and 3 we explored the essential trauma-sensitive yoga (TSY) practices of interoception and choice making. Now the key question before us is, what do we do once we feel something and/or choose to do something? For many traumatized people it is one huge challenge to notice a body feeling, another huge challenge to choose what to do with their bodies once they feel something and, perhaps the greatest challenge of all, to actually take an action based on what they feel in their bodies. To make this leap from *feeling something* and/or *choosing something* to *doing something*, one must trust one's body as a useful, functional thing. But, as we have seen, to be traumatized is to live in a body that is more likely to feel useless and ineffectual. Immediately we can sense the dilemma. A traumatized body has been chronically acted on; it has rarely, if at all, been the agent. In fact, it is possible to suggest that in order to survive the kinds of ordeals that our clients have been through it really doesn't make sense to the organism (and I use that word purposefully as I did in Chapter 3 because this may well not be a conscious choice, especially for people who are born into and/or grow up in abusive, chaotic environments) to continue to use energy at exerting its own will if it always fails. Perhaps energy is better spent just trying to survive. In order to heal from trauma, we must begin to do more than survive. We must reclaim our body as a successful agent of action and change.

## Action, intentional action, and effective action

Taking action is a description of a larger paradigm, which has three components that I would like to describe. Once I have described them, I will resort to the term *taking action* but it will be understood that it represents some or all of the three components (as we will see, it is not required that all three components be satisfied in order for action taking to have therapeutic value). The three components are as follows:

- **Action:** Something you do with your body; something purely motoric
- **Intentional action:** Something you do with your body that is purposeful (based on an idea or feeling)
- **Effective action:** Something you do with your body that you notice results in feeling better physically

### Action
Every yoga form offers an opportunity for action, that is, doing something with your body, though every action does not have to be intentional or effective. Consider the case example that opened this chapter. Sam's action is to stand

up. That is a purely motoric thing, which results in his moving his body from sitting to standing. There is a place in TSY and trauma treatment in general for simply acting, that is, doing something with the body, even if the action is not based on any idea. This happens when we choose to move our arms in one way and not another, for no particular reason. This phenomenon is purely motoric and doesn't require any forethought or analysis. Just acting could, under certain circumstances, like in the context of a yoga form, be very therapeutic for some clients.

## Intentional action

However, consider the example of Sam that opened this chapter. While Sam takes an action when he stands up there are other things going on that factor into our overall understanding of taking action within the context of TSY. Before standing, Sam noticed some discomfort in his back and he told the TSY facilitator what he was feeling. The facilitator's response is the invitation to stand. So not only did Sam do something motoric but it was also preceded by his awareness of discomfort in his back and an invitation from the TSY facilitator. Once the facilitator made the invitation to stand, it became an idea to Sam (maybe an idea that standing might make his back feel better, we don't really know, but at least an idea like "do I want to keep sitting or do I want to stand?"). Therefore, even though the idea to stand is presented at first as an invitation, Sam's act of standing becomes an intentional action because it was done on purpose (based, ultimately, on some idea and/or body feeling of his own). In this equation, an action has to be purposeful to be considered intentional but it can originate from either the client or the TSY facilitator. As long as the client has a choice and is not compelled to act, he is the "owner" of the action once he engages in it.

Actions that are planned and carried out on purpose we call intentional actions. These occur any time we decide to do something based on what we feel: "my back is tight: I will stand" or "I would rather stand than sit right now" or "my legs feel strong: I want to use them to stand up." Clearly, taking action based on these kinds of awarenesses can be very beneficial in the context of trauma treatment. In fact, this may be a very good definition of empowerment, which, as we have seen, Judith Herman encourages us to make a central part of trauma treatment.

It is also useful to compare action, taking action, and the other key part of TSY methodology discussed in Chapter 3: making choices. Action and intentional action as I have presented them are both the result of some kind of choice. More to the point, I would suggest that actions may be choice based or may not be (there are such phenomena as unconscious actions), but intentional actions are always choice based. By its very definition, an intentional action is one that requires a purpose, and purpose requires choice (I need to know I have options in order to do something purposefully). An intentional action is one that we choose to take no matter how obscure our purpose may be (we may know for sure what we want to accomplish by our action or we may have only a vague idea). Our work with TSY is to help our clients take as many intentional actions as possible.

### Effective action

The third and final aspect of taking action is effective action, and it is different: it stands alone. Notice the next couple of things that happened after Sam took his intentional action. First, the facilitator asks the question "How does your back feel now?" to which Sam replies, "Hey, it feels a lot better." Assuming that Sam is reporting what he actually feels (which may not always be the case, as sometimes people will tell you what they think you want to hear), this is a key piece to the puzzle of trauma treatment and is, in fact, inviting an act of interoception. Sam made a choice (to stand) and then he took an intentional action (standing on purpose) but when he notices that his back now feels better (interoception) it is at this point we can say that Sam has taken an *effective action*. So an effective action is not the action or intentional action itself but rather the action or the intentional action *plus* the experience of noticing that the action we have taken makes us feel better (notice that an action can end up being effective even if it wasn't intentional: "I just stood up for some rea-son and then noticed how much better my back felt. I hadn't even realized how sore my back was!"). We cannot determine whether or not an action is effective until we have taken it. In Sam's case, to check out the effectiveness of his action even further, he decided to try it again and this time to notice the muscles he used to make it happen. He was able to identify and feel specific muscles that he used in order to stand and then, one last time, to acknowledge that his back felt better. In an attempt to characterize an internal process, I would suggest that what happened was Sam noticed he could feel muscles in his legs, which he could use to help him move from sitting to standing; as a result, by using his leg muscles on purpose, his back felt better. (This sounds a little simplistic but it is the kind of process we hope will become as conscious as possible to our clients. They may not connect all of the dots but even a couple would be very helpful in the overall process of trauma treatment.) Through this process of taking action, Sam began to solidify new truths within his organism that his body is feel-able, has agency, is effectual and capable of feeling more than one thing, and can do something on purpose to change the way he feels. This process, after all, is how a healthy organism functions.

Please note, however, that in the context of TSY, as I have stated before, it would have been an equally valid trauma treatment had Sam noticed that his back still felt the same or even worse after standing. It is not primarily the fact that Sam's action was effective that made this process a useful part of treatment. It was the fact that Sam was able to interocept, make a choice, and take action. It is not required or expected that people feel better as a result of any of this: it is just one possibility among many. Taking action in TSY just allows for the possibility of perceiving change but it does not require any perceived change to be for the better. If, for example, Sam felt more pain in his back when standing it would be possible for him and the TSY facilitator to try other yoga forms like a gentle twist or a seated forward fold, for example (see Chapter 8 for these and other possibilities). Perhaps Sam would find that one of these forms relieved his back pain; if not, if the whole thing became overwhelming for that day, he could stop TSY altogether and move on to something else (like some kind of verbal processing if the

TSY facilitator is a qualified clinician). The bottom line is that some clients will practice the motoric aspect of taking action, others will engage in the intentional aspect of taking action, and some will notice when an action is effective. With TSY we just want to make all of these possibilities available as often as possible and as long as they are tolerable to our clients.

Our experience working with people who have experienced complex trauma is that most often this process is disrupted at some point along the way: people may not feel the back tightness in the first place or, if they do, they may not have any idea what to do with it or, if they do have an idea and make a choice about what to do, they may not be able to carry out their choice. As we have seen, the reasons behind this disruption may be neurophysiological (less activity in the interoceptive pathways of the brain as a result of trauma) or relational (learning through experience with traumatic relationships that it is safer to not feel oneself or to not express vulnerability or to not trust one's intuition to act) or something else but, for our purposes, the underlying reason doesn't matter so much. The fact is that, in our work with trauma survivors, it is very common for people to experience one or more of these kinds of disruptions and that this is a large part of why it is so difficult to live with the impact of trauma: we can't feel our bodies, we can't make choices about what to do with our bodies, and/or we have difficulty taking action of any kind, especially actions based on what we feel in our bodies. With the example above, Sam may have begun rebuilding his frontal lobe or he may be learning through his relationship with the TSY facilitator that it is safe and acceptable to feel something, to express it to another person, and to make a choice about what to do and so on. As of the publication of this book, though we can speculate based on the evidence we have begun to accumulate, we just do not know the underlying mechanisms of TSY to a definitive empirical degree. But one thing is for sure: Sam is having experiences with his body that are different from experiences of trauma. He specifically feels his back, he chooses to do something about it, he acts on his choice, and, in this case, he notices a positive outcome.

## Integrating interoception, making choices, and taking action

I consider some combination of interoception, choice making, and action taking to be at the heart of TSY. They do not have to happen all at once for a session to be considered successful, but we, as TSY facilitators, should always be oriented to ways we can bring them into the process. In my example above, I identified action (and especially intentional action) with choice, and effective action with interoception. Figure 4.1 represents a way to bring them all together.

Figure 4.1 begins with noticing what we feel in our bodies (introception), which leads to making a choice based on what we feel in our bodies, which is followed by acting either intentionally (purposefully) or not (purely motorically) and ends back with interoception, which determines whether or not the action was effective. This process represents a fundamental shift from a way of being whereby we are uncontrollably living in a body that belongs to the past (trauma) to living in a body that exists in the present and that can change from one state or experience to another. All of these components are the opposite of trauma in the way that I have defined it. Figure 4.1 gives a general way to understand the process but it is a linear model, which implies a rigid approach. Therefore, while it may be helpful in some circumstances to think linearly, let's consider another model that opens up the possibilities, as depicted in Figure 4.2.

In Figure 4.2, the process is not linear but circular and can begin at any point marked on the circle. For example, an experience could begin with interoception, which may have been the case for Sam (noticing his back was sore), which leads to a choice (the idea to stand), which leads to an intentional action (standing on purpose), which then led to further interoception (noticing his back felt better), which allows Sam to understand the action as an effective one. It would also be possible for a cycle like this to begin with an action like standing up, then lead to interoception like noticing your knee hurts when you stand, which may lead to other choices and/or actions. The broad suggestion here is that as

$$\text{Interoception} \Rightarrow \text{choice} \Rightarrow \frac{\text{action}\ (\text{motoric})}{\text{intentional action}\ (\text{purposeful})} \Rightarrow \frac{\text{interoception}}{(\text{effective action})}$$

**Figure 4.1.** A linear depiction of integrating interoception, making choices, and taking actions

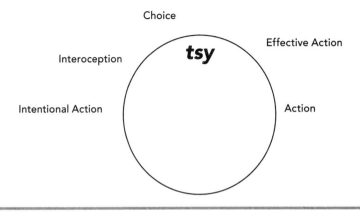

**Figure 4.2.** A circular depiction of integrating interoception, making choices, and taking actions

long as we are engaged in either interocepting, choosing, and acting either motorically or purposefully (or some combination of these dynamics), we are not stuck in a trauma paradigm. We experience new possibilities with regard to our bodies that are not the same as typical traumatic body experiences like not feeling, not knowing what to do, and not knowing how to make bad feelings change. Or, as Bessel van der Kolk has said, "Once patients become aware of their sensations and action tendencies they can set about . . . exploring new ways of engaging with potential sources of mastery" (van der Kolk, 2006, p. 13).

Once a client begins to develop some level of comfort and familiarity with interoception, choice, and taking action, then the two of you together may want to experiment with increasing the *complexity* and the *depth* of the experience. Yoga forms like those presented throughout this book offer myriad opportunities to feel what you feel, make choices, and take actions. The continued challenge for the TSY facilitator is not to turn these experiences into stories about the past (i.e., ways we acted or did not act previously) or the future (i.e., ways we might act in the future) but to keep the focus solely on what is happening right now. In the broader course of therapy there certainly may be time and space for talking about the past or the future but TSY is an opportunity to focus completely on having and noticing experiences that are happening in the here and now and to experiment with interacting with what you feel in your body by taking actions.

## Conclusions

Like interoception and choice making, the practice of taking action is a key part of the TSY methodology. However, like everything else we have encountered, the kind of action we are going for is the self-motivated kind: the kind we choose for ourselves. Because of the context of complex trauma treatment there will be times when the facilitator will need to make the idea of an action available to a client but this is when it is critically important that they are committed to not commanding or coercing. Every idea, every cue, is presented as a genuine invitation for the client. The action becomes valuable only if it is self-motivated and/or based on interoception. If the action is taken as a result of external coercion, it is at best a waste of time and at worst retraumatizing. The encouragement is to proceed cautiously but to give as many opportunities as possible for your clients to use the yoga forms as ways to take self-motivated actions.

We have established interoception, choice making, and action taking as the foundational aspects of TSY methodology but there are some other vitally important qualities of the practice that we can look at throughout the next three chapters, beginning with an investigation of the present moment and how it bears on the treatment of complex trauma.

# 5

# BEING PRESENT

THE GROUP FOR TEENS HAD MET ON THE INPATIENT UNIT
of the hospital for several months. The format included both
a trauma-sensitive yoga (TSY) portion (for 15 minutes at the
beginning) and a more narrative, trauma processing portion
(for 45 minutes). The facilitator was trained in both TSY and
clinical psychology. One evening they were standing in their
socks on the wood floor and experimenting with noticing
their feet on the ground. The facilitator invited everyone to
try two different ways of noticing: the first was to look and
see with their eyes and the second was "to feel." In order to
feel their feet on the ground they were encouraged to experiment with shifting their weight from side to side and from
heel to toe. The question was then directly posed by the facilitator: "Do you feel your feet on the ground?" At first, Sheryl,
a young woman with a significant history of childhood
trauma and currently in state custody for a violent crime,
couldn't remember anyone ever having asked her that question before. In fact she couldn't remember ever asking herself
a question like that, let alone being invited by someone else
to notice anything about what her body felt like. It actually
seemed weird as she started to think about it. But she smiled.
She recalled that she had been doing TSY like this for a few

months and actually words like "do you feel your feet on the ground?" had been said a lot during the sessions but Sheryl, for some reason, just never thought they applied to her. The words never felt like they were for her. For some reason it was like she was hearing them, really hearing them, for the first time. She became curious and interested in what she could feel with her feet. She moved from the wood floor to the rug, and she noticed she could feel a difference in texture. She moved from the rug back to the wood floor, and she noticed she could feel a difference in temperature. For a few moments, Sheryl was totally involved with, completely transfixed by, what she could feel with her own feet.

## What does it mean to be present?

In this chapter I focus on why the idea of "presence" is such a central concept to TSY and how it can be facilitated. In order to give some context for our understanding of this very important part of TSY, I need to bring up some different ways of thinking about being present. But first, to get us started, I would like to invite you to try a practice.

The investigation of feeling your feet making contact with the ground, as depicted in the case story above, is a fundamental TSY practice of being present. If you would like to try this yourself, the invitation is to either stand or sit in a chair and, as you are able, bring your feet flat to the floor. (It is important to point out that feeling your feet on the ground is by no means the only way to practice being present. If this one isn't available, readers could experiment with feeling their hands making contact with a surface or practice bringing awareness to wherever their body is making contact with a surface beneath it. The important thing in this case is to figure out where your body is in contact with a surface and to investigate feeling that connection.) Please take a moment to notice that your feet are on the floor. One way to notice might be to look and see; another way to notice is to feel. In order to feel your feet on the floor, you may want to experiment with either shifting from side to side if you are standing or tapping your heels and toes if you are sitting. You may notice some sensation, some feeling underneath your feet when you shift around or tap your heels and toes. Perhaps there are some other things you can do that help you feel your feet on the floor, like shuffling or sliding your feet around a bit. In any case, if you like, give yourself a moment to experiment with feeling your feet on the ground.

Though I will describe the mechanisms involved in this practice of being present later in this chapter, for now, notice that being present in terms of TSY is a *body* thing and not a *thinking* thing. In order to put our TSY practice of being present in some context, let's briefly look at how being present—and the concept of the "present moment"—has emerged recently in the field of mental health and wellness.

## A new age movement

The concept of "being present" became a very powerful idea in my cultural milieu during the second half of the twentieth century. A whole genre of popular literature since the 1950s has been devoted largely to the exploration of being present epitomized in such works as Ram Dass's book *Be Here Now*; Jon Kabat-Zinn's *Wherever You Go, There You Are*;

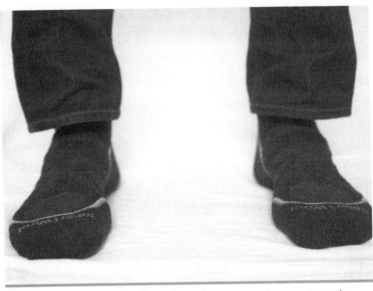

**Figure 5.1.** Feet-on-the-Ground exercise—a present-moment practice.

and Eckhart Tolle's *The Power of Now.* These books have sold millions of copies collectively and represent a very powerful strand of modern spiritual and psychological inquiry that is often referred to as the new age movement. In general, the kinds of experiences that the new age movement associates with being present involve some aspect of a thinking process. Being present is often described as a realization that occurs within the mind, which doesn't necessarily have anything to do with something we feel in our body. In fact, this kind of being present is also tellingly referred to as *mindfulness.* Of mindfulness, Kabat-Zinn says, "It has to do with examining who we are, with questioning our view of the world and our place in it, and with cultivating some appreciation for the fullness of each moment we are alive. Most of all, it has to do with being in touch" (1994, p. 3).

Immediately, based on the Feet-on-the-Ground exercise, we can see that this is a very different kind of experience of being present than what we aim for with TSY. With the new age movement, we have a focus on being present that starts with the activity of the mind versus an experience that starts with the activity of the body, which is the TSY perspective. Nevertheless, though it is not within the scope of this book to go into any methodological detail related to the ways that Kabat-Zinn and others suggest one go about the practice of being present, it is important for the thesis of this book to note that the new age movement did a great deal of good in terms of bringing to popular consciousness the idea that being present is something that one could practice in order to increase their quality of life. While aspects of mindfulness had been deeply integrated into many world cultures for millennia, these authors carved out space within the Western zeitgeist where being present could be talked about and investigated and practiced by ordinary people in a non-religious context and this has proven in many ways to be a tremendous service: one that TSY does benefit from for sure.

## A clinical understanding

Along with the development of being present within the new age context, there was a simultaneous investigation of the phenomenon within the clinical community: in particular, the clinical community devoted to understanding trauma. One way for us to understand the role of being present in the clinical milieu involves the understanding of traumatic memory as opposed to nontraumatic memory. There is a complex story to be told here but it starts with the current understanding that nontraumatic memories are dealt with differently in the organism than traumatic ones. Most important for us, the parts of the brain that are normally involved in the storage and processing of memory, like the prefrontal cortex, are impacted by trauma (Samuelson, 2011). Instead of being managed primarily by the executive part of the brain, traumatic memories are dealt with primarily by the emotional part of the brain, or limbic system (Samuelson, 2011). Importantly, researchers have indicated that the way traumatic memory is stored and processed is not a pathology in and of itself but rather a sign of health in that traumatic memories are, in real ways, more important than others due to their potential impact on survival (Morey, Dolcos, et al., 2009). The pathology, or the suffering of the individual, is not due to the way the organism handles traumatic memory in the first place but rather in the way that traumatic memory lingers over time and the way it impacts future experiences. Researchers like R. A. Morey (2008, 2009) and Rachel Yehuda (1995) have demonstrated that traumatic memories crowd out nontraumatic ones and make it very difficult for traumatized people to learn new things and have new experiences. One final piece of very pertinent, more recent, research into memory indicates that normal memories, sometimes called declarative memories (those that are organized mostly by the frontal lobe), can change over time (Bridge & Paller, 2012). I believe that it can be speculated that the ability for memory to be somewhat fluid and not rigid may suggest a certain aspect of health: namely that our memories might not be as important to who we are as we think. In contrast, Bessel van der Kolk has called traumatic memories "timeless and unmodified by further experience" (van der Kolk, 1994, p. 259). This "timelessness" to traumatic memory is presented as anathema to "further experience" and therefore we can understand it as a mutually exclusive dichotomy: if memories are timeless, they do not allow space for new experiences. In this paradigm, in order to have new experiences, we need to be present and available for them so we can understand traumatic memory as in some way making it difficult for us to be present and available for new experiences. This is why figuring out ways to be present, to actually experience the present moment, is of such central importance to the treatment of trauma.

Van der Kolk summarized this entire conundrum when he wrote that traumatized people "have difficulty with being fully engaged in the present" (van der Kolk, 2006, p. 4). This idea that not being able to be present (what he had earlier referred to as being stuck in the timelessness of traumatic memory) is right at the heart of the suffering associated with trauma comes up again and again in van der Kolk's work over time. Interestingly, while van der Kolk makes his statements regarding being present with particular regard to brain research and clinical treatment of trauma, and not as an existential phenomenon like that posited by those in the new age movement, the implications were the same: people who have difficulty being present will suffer; *traumatized people suffer more because they have a more difficult time than nontraumatized people in being present.*

From the perspectives of both the new age movement and the clinical work of van der Kolk and others, not being present is a problem that must be reckoned with on the one hand in order to live a happy life and on the other in order to heal trauma. What is revealed by these two perspectives is that in a certain sense the playing field is leveled. That is, being present is framed as both an aspect of trauma treatment but also as something that will benefit all of us: traumatized and nontraumatized alike. True, the stakes are higher for those who experience complex trauma but we, as both client and TSY facilitator, share something in common; we can both practice being present and we will both benefit from it. So, as we continue, I invite readers to keep this commonality in mind even as we specifically investigate how being present functions as part of treatment for complex trauma. It seems very clear based on the research indicated above and much more that trauma involves being stuck in the past (in part as aspects of traumatic memory being played out in the body) and treatment involves being able to be present. Once we understand how difficult it is for traumatized people to be present and how painful it is to always be oriented to the past, we must ask ourselves, as caregivers, how can I make the present moment available to my client?

## What does it mean to be present as a treatment for complex trauma?

We have seen that being present can be understood as a clinical challenge for trauma sufferers whose ability to store and retrieve memories has been affected, but there are some other important perspectives to consider. To take this next step I propose that we declare some simplified boundaries on our inquiry with the following two questions: Is being present a cognitive experience, an idea, something we can think about like "I am present"? Or is it something expe-riential, something we feel in our bodies? If these are the only two options, and I suggest that they are (though not necessarily mutually exclusive), then consider the possibil-ity that one could have the thought "I am present" without any experiential basis. In other words, how do you know if you are present if your only point of reference is a thought? I could think "I am present" right now as I sit here writ-ing these words but I could also just as easily be thinking about a trip to Amsterdam and think "what will the weather be like when I go to Amsterdam next month?" Maybe I'll start to think about the winding streets I have walked down before; the smell of the air; the sound of the bicycles speed-ing past. While my body is here in a cafe in Cambridge, Massachusetts, I use my brain to think myself to Amsterdam in the same way that Dorothy uses her brain to bring herself back to Kansas through her mantra "there's no place like home." Though Dorothy actually awoke in her Kansas bed, surely many of our thinking experiences involve things that do not actually happen: I do not expect that I will blink and open my eyes in Amsterdam! What does this mean for the implications of using any thought as the basis for having a present-moment experience? At least it is suspect. With TSY we are interested in what is *actually* happening and what is actually happening *always* involves the body.

Though we started our investigation of what it means to be present with the new age movement that began in the 1950s the investigation of being present goes back even farther in the Western tradition to the beginnings of Greek intellectual history. Sometime around 500 BCE, the Greek philosopher

Heraclitus said, "You could not step twice into the same river; for other waters are ever flowing onto you." This sounds a lot like the current research into memory, which indicates that memories change with time and experience. But Heraclitus is also making a very interesting statement about what it means to be present: it is literally not actually possible to step into the exact same water molecules twice for they move too fast! Further, of utmost importance to TSY, the experience that Heraclitus describes is not something that starts as an idea, but rather with a body experience: stepping into that river. It is an experience that requires the ability to interact, through the body as intermediary, with what is happening right now and what is happening is always changing; it's always new.

Here we can consider the understanding of trauma that we are developing; to be traumatized means not being able to take on new experiences. For traumatized people, Heraclitus's water (and, therefore, water molecules) has completely, and unnaturally, stagnated and every time they step into the river it is the same; the river (the trauma or traumatic memory) is "timeless" in the words of van der Kolk. Another way to frame this is to say that, for a traumatized person, being present becomes an experience of always "standing" in trauma. Trauma bends the natural flow of time back into itself where new experiences become less and less possible and the only experience actually left is trauma. Imagine if in a cruel twist of fate, being present came to mean always experiencing the horror of trauma: who would want to be present under those conditions? None of us would want that. Yet this largely describes the experience of those with complex trauma: they are stuck always and (seemingly) forever in it.

Another way to frame this is that traumatized people are alive and being introduced to new experiences like everyone else; it's just that by far (really, beyond compare) the most compelling experience of their lives has been trauma and therefore they end up experiencing the same thing over and over again while others get to move on and have new experiences. Ultimately, trauma is an experience of not being able to experience anything new. We are starting to add nuance to the understanding of being present; along with the importance of body experience we can add the ability to experience new things as fundamental. Back to Heraclitus: "the only constant is change." For traumatized people, the only constant is trauma. Trauma, understood as an entity, has usurped the power of change and installed itself in its place. The work of TSY involves learning that being present is to experience what is happening in the body and that what is happening in the body is always experienced as new; it is never the same. Before we move into the most important thing, how we can actually practice being present, I would like to note that our discussion has just now circled back to a previous concept that I alerted readers would come up many times in this book.

## Interoception: An addendum

In TSY, when we practice being present, we start with the body. Being present is always a body experience. We are not interested in the thought "I am present" because, as we have seen above, thoughts can be things that are not happening. From this perspective, trauma is not primarily a problem of what I am thinking but a problem of what I am feeling in my body: either not feeling anything or feeling stuck forever in a painful, tortured, broken body that will never change. Again, van der Kolk says that because of the way they are stored, "It is possible that traumatic memories then could emerge, not in the distorted fashion of ordinary recall, but as affect states, somatic sensations or as visual images" (van der Kolk, 1994, p. 259). (As a brief aside it is worth pausing and noticing that the implication here, which is important to TSY, is that in some ways traumatic memories, which are imprinted with reliable somatic detail on the organism, are more reliable than declarative memories, which are prone to change over time. In this way, we are dealing with reality and we will be better at helping traumatized people if we acknowledge that fact.) Also, traumatized people experience their bodies as stuck in or constantly reactive to the trauma because parts of the brain that allow us to feel the present state of our body, our viscera, are damaged (van der Kolk, 2006). Our work is to help people find ways to have new body experiences right now that can effectively replace the constant replay button of trauma.

So now we come back to the practice example that opened this chapter. Can you feel where your feet are? Can you feel the surface underneath you? Or, as another example, if you extend one leg, do you feel the big muscles on top of your leg engage in some way? There are so many things happening in your body right now (or things you could purposefully make happen) that provide a vast array of opportunities to practice being present. Readers will notice that what I describe here in terms of being present already has a word for it that acts like a touchstone throughout this book: *interoception*. So we now have an addendum to our previous definitions of interoception to work with: being present. More specifically, being present is when one's body experience and one's neurobiological experience are aligned. That is, when what is happening in my body (my feet are on the ground or my leg muscle is contracting) and what is happening in my brain (the associated neural circuitry that we might call *I feel my feet on the ground* or *I feel my leg muscle contracting,* or *the pathways of interoception*) are both oriented to the same thing. The kind of experience of being present that we are aiming for with TSY involves doing something with the body and feeling it. Do a gentle seated twist and feel the space around your rib cage. Gently lift your chin and feel sensation in the front of your throat. And, indeed, place your feet on the ground and notice the texture or the temperature or the feeling of pressure under your feet. The work of TSY is to invite our clients to experiment with various yoga forms and then to notice what they feel so that they can have new, present-moment experiences that are, in effect, not trauma. To borrow from the language of Heraclitus, the river begins to flow again.

## TSY practices that emphasize being present

Now let's turn our attention more explicitly to some practices that encourage being present. The example I brought up at the beginning of this chapter is a seminal practice of being present but I would like to give a few other options. I indicated earlier that some clients will not be able to feel their feet on the ground. This can be true for various reasons, including the neurophysiological impact of trauma, or perhaps you are working with war veterans or survivors of physical violence that has left them without one or both feet. In any case the suggestion is to not force anything and if for any reason your client is not able to use their feet as a way to have a body experience your work is to help them find a part of their body that they do have access to.

In terms of practicing being present we can think of the body as simply a vehicle for interoceptive experiences (I would be the first to argue that the body is more than this but for the purposes of this chapter we can compartmentalize a bit if it's helpful). Work with your client to find a part of the body that is feel-able for her. In one case I worked with a small group of three teenagers with significant trauma histories who were hospitalized for experiencing some psychotic features related to their trauma histories. We did TSY together once a week and on one occasion we experimented with feeling our feet on the ground. For some reason, all three had a very difficult time with this and became upset about it, so I quickly tried something else. My intention was to remain focused on a body-based practice of being present. We were sitting at a table with several things on it: pencils, paper, glue bottles, staplers, cups (it was a modified classroom). I invited everyone to pick up different objects from the table and to experiment with feeling any sensation in their bodies associated with picking up the objects. We started to notice we could feel different textures and temperatures with our hands; we were on to something!

Next I invited us to notice if we could feel different muscles in our arms depending on the weight of the object. This became a fun and interesting activity, as opposed to frustrating and upsetting like the Feet-on-the-Ground exercise had been, and we noticed several different muscles in our arms that we could feel as we began to pick up the heavier objects; someone even noticed he could feel some back muscles that he was using, which I hadn't cued! This exercise was not what I had originally planned and it may not look like the kind of yoga that was happening at the yoga studio down the street, but it was a core TSY practice because we were doing things with our bodies and noticing what we felt; we were practicing being present.

Another of my favorite exercises for being present involves using big leg muscles. If your client is willing and able (or if you would like to try this yourself right now) you can invite him to stand and then to bend his knees a little bit. Once you are standing and bending your knees a little bit (like a skier would) you may notice a feeling in the big muscles at the top of your legs. These muscles are called quadriceps and when you stand and bend your knees like this they contract (they draw in toward a center point in order to support the structure of your body in this form). All you need to do is to offer an invitation like "If you like, feel free to stand and bend your knees a little bit. When you do this you may notice a feeling in the top of your legs." (It is better not to add any adjectives, if possible, like muscles *tighten* or muscles *strengthen* as this can easily become manipulative.) If it is helpful, you can point directly to the top of your legs as a way to indicate where sensation might be experienced, but then let your client have a few seconds to practice feeling something. At this point, especially if it is in a one-to-one session or a small group, I often ask directly, "Do you notice a feeling in the top of your legs?" (Readers: Please notice that asking a direct question like this is what I have earlier referred to as a high dose of interoception so please be sure you know your client well if you choose to try this. Otherwise you could just let your invitation to notice any feeling in the top of the legs stand alone.) Feeling big muscles (or any muscles) actually do something like contract, extend, or rest is a present-moment experience, and every yoga form in this book will allow for opportunities of this kind.

## Conclusions

Being present is something to practice feeling in the body. It is related directly to interoception and is another non-cognitive experience; we do not ask our clients to imagine being present or to make a story out of any body experience they notice. For example, if your client feels her feet on the ground do not ask her to relate that experience to her previously expressed distress at not being able to feel her body at all. Just let the experience stand alone and, in a sense, speak for itself. Like everything else in TSY, we do not coerce our clients into having present-moment experiences, we simply make some opportunities available, within the context of treatment, for them to notice what they feel and thereby have present-moment experiences.

While being present, like everything else, is a body-oriented undertaking, there are more qualities to the embodied experience that have bearing on trauma treatment and are important to investigate. So let's keep our focus on the body as we consider our muscle dynamics in more detail.

# 6

# MUSCLE DYNAMICS AND BREATHWORK

A SMALL GROUP OF WAR VETERANS HAD BEEN MEETING TO do trauma-sensitive yoga (TSY) every week for several years. The veterans had various physical injuries (and no small amount of medications being taken for both pain and psychiatric conditions) so the decision was made early on to stick with chair-based yoga. On one occasion, they experimented with some core strength in the chairs by leaning back a little and holding themselves at a slight recline (see Figure 6.1).

The TSY facilitator invited them to notice what muscles they were using to hold themselves in this position. After a few breaths, they returned back up to a neutral position, the Seated Mountain Form, and the invitation was to notice what muscles felt less intense as they moved out of the reclined position. They did this together several times and one of the group participants said, "I feel my stomach muscles." Someone else said, "If I lean back further, those muscles feel more intense." Someone else in the small group said, "I notice a feeling in my back."

At this point, the TSY instructor invited them all, if they

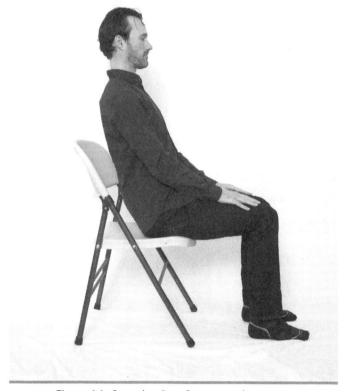

**Figure 6.1.** Seated recline: Core strength exercise.

were interested in making it a little more intense, to lift one leg off the ground and notice what happened to the muscles in their leg. Somebody noticed the muscles on the top of their leg got "tighter." Someone else said, "When I do this [lifts one leg], it feels like my stomach muscles get harder, more firm." Several others experimented with lifting one leg a little and noticing what they felt. After a few breaths they all sat back upright in a more neutral position. The TSY facilitator asked, "Do you feel your muscles get a little less intense?" Somebody said, "My leg muscles feel a little softer" and someone else in the room said, "Yeah, I feel my stomach muscles get less intense but I couldn't really feel it at first—it took a few seconds."

## What are muscle dynamics?

As we have seen throughout this book, everything that we do with TSY involves the body. Muscle dynamics are the things about our muscles that we can feel, those things that we can interocept. As will become clear in this chapter, there are many things we can do with our bodies that allow us to have dynamic experiences, including one of the things we each do every moment of every day: breathe.

While we do not have to have an in-depth understanding of physiology in order to help people feel their muscle dynamics, here are a few useful terms to become acquainted with (readers interested in a more thorough understanding of muscle dynamics may wish to consult any number of good books on physiology, including Coulter, 2001):

> **Strengthen/contract:** Muscles often feel stronger (get more firm, more engaged) when they contract (draw together toward a midpoint). A contraction is happening in Figure 6.1, for example, when our stomach muscles (more precisely, muscle fibers) draw toward a midpoint in order to support our body in this reclined form.
>
> **Stretch/lengthen:** When we extend a muscle, we lengthen it as in the form called Back and Shoulder Stretch,

Variation 2 in Chapter 8. This is an example of stretching/lengthening back muscles.

**Rest:** For our purposes, this is when we allow muscles to not do anything. It may not be immediately obvious but this is also feel-able. For an example of how you might bring an experience of muscles resting into the TSY session, see Figure 8.29.

With TSY, you can give your client a chance to feel any or all of the above. Like everything else, some dynamics will be more feel-able than others and the work is to help your clients find what they have access to in their bodies and to build from there.

## Noticing intensity shifts

Another way to feel muscles is to experiment with noticing intensity shifts within muscles; that is, start by feeling a muscle or group of muscles do one thing and then shift dynamically to an opposite state. For example, one way to do this begins with the core strength exercise from our case example above and also depicted in Figure 6.1. Readers may wish to try this exercise themselves.

If you would like to experiment with this form, the invitation is to start by sitting comfortably tall. Maybe just pause for a moment and experiment with sitting up in a way where you are relatively comfortable and your spine is tall. When you are ready, you can recline (lean back) slightly and then hold at some point. Feel free to use Figure 6.1 as a guide but how much you actually recline is totally up to you: it's your choice. You may wish to investigate this reclined action for a moment and find an angle that feels comfortable to you. When you recline and hold at some angle, do you feel some muscles in your body start to engage? Maybe the abdominal muscles, stomach muscles, core muscles become a little bit more intense? If you like, hang out and breathe (more on breath in TSY later in this chapter) in this reclined form for a few seconds, noticing that the muscles you feel become more intense or more active (or more firm, if a tactile cue is more helpful). The other possibility is that you might not feel anything in this form and that is ok too. Remember that the expectation is not to feel something in particular but just to notice when you do feel or when you do not feel anything.

When you are ready, you may wish to sit back up straight or to even lean forward a little bit, as in Figure 6.2. When you sit up straight or lean forward a little bit you might feel a change in your core muscles. When you sit upright or lean forward a little bit, your core muscles go back toward a more neutral state. In other words, the very muscles that became very activated when you reclined may become less activated when you sit up straight and possibly less active still if you lean forward. You may feel a dynamic change in your core muscles as you move between these various forms. If you like, you can try this whole sequence again—reclining and holding, sitting up straight, and/or leaning forward—and experiment with noticing intensity shifts in your muscles.

Chapter 8 offers various yoga forms that you and your clients can experiment with in order to find opportunities to feel some intensity shifts within muscles.

## Muscle dynamics add something new: Purpose

In developing TSY over time I have benefited from many conversations with clinicians, neuroscientists, and fellow yoga teachers. These discussions sometimes include anecdotal observations based on our professional experiences and occasionally those observations turn into something practical. One such anecdotal observation is that our traumatized clients often experience a lack of purpose as they navigate through life. The kind of purpose I am referring to is not equated with meaning (i.e., what is the purpose of my life?) but is rather equated with action, as in I am doing something with my body on purpose (walking, running, reaching, etc.) toward a desired result. For people who are not severely traumatized, the suggestion is that actions are usually connected to a desired result: I am getting myself to the gym because I want to get stronger; I am walking because I want to get to work; I am marching in this demonstration because I want my government to change something; I am reaching for something on the top shelf at the grocery store because I want that particular food. Here is a depiction of the relationship between action and purpose:

> Purpose    =    I do [fill in the action]
> because I want [fill in the desired result].

Even during times when we act without a strong conscious conceptualization of the outcome we desire, we are still frequently engaged in acting with a purpose, albeit sub- or unconsciously.

The implication is that, for traumatized people, action is very often disconnected from a desired outcome and therefore from purpose itself. As a yoga teacher I sometimes see this in the way a student chronically moves through the world very slowly, eyes down, breath shallow, shoulders rounded forward (again, not to say that there is one physical stance that indicates complex trauma but just to illustrate my personal experience with what I have interpreted as a sense

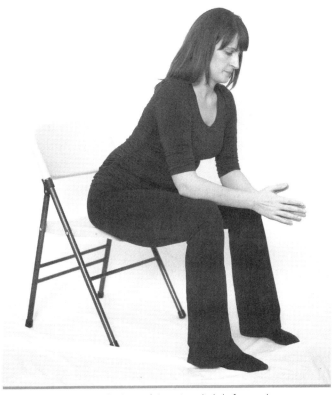

**Figure 6.2.** Seated: Leaning slightly forward.

of purposelessness in some of my students). Bessel van der Kolk refers to this phenomenon when he says, "People who suffer from PTSD seem to lose their way in the world" (van der Kolk, 2006, p. 4). When our action is decoupled from a desired result, we lack purpose or, more colorfully, we have lost our way in the world.

$$\frac{\text{No purpose}}{\text{[lost our way in the world]}} = \frac{\text{I do [fill in the action]}}{\text{because [?]}}.$$

Why do I act or move through the world? There is still action: we still walk here and there and move through grocery stores but we do so without purpose; we are going through the motions. With TSY we can begin to restore purpose to our actions. Specifically, using muscle dynamics, we can begin the investigation that what happens to my muscles is not random but something I can be consciously in charge of.

While at times it will be enough to just feel our muscles become more and less intense, there is also the possibility of noticing that these feelings are happening because we are doing something. We *are in charge of these dynamics (and, therefore, feelings in our muscles) and we can change them on purpose.*

Your client purposefully creates the intensity in her stomach muscles when she reclines and holds. She purposefully rests her stomach muscles when she moves from that reclined position back to neutral, or when she leans slightly forward. She is purposefully creating the feeling (muscles stretching) in the side of her body when she reaches one arm up toward the ceiling and leans a little bit to the opposite side in a side stretch. You, as the TSY facilitator, can pick opportunities to make "purpose" an explicit theme as you explore yoga forms by saying something like "notice that you can make these muscles in your body more or less intense *on purpose*." Or "You are in charge of the feeling you are creating in your body right now; you can make it more or less intense." The encouragement is to intentionally use the word "purpose" (or some equivalent) from time to time connected with an actual body experience within a yoga form in order to give your client a chance to do something with her body with a desired outcome. While we cannot attribute a desired outcome to an action from the outside, we can give our client some space to do this for herself (i.e., "I will lift my leg a few inches higher because I want to feel strength in those muscles" or "I will lower my leg because I do not want to feel those muscles right now").

The added value to trauma treatment comes through noticing that *you* are creating these feelings in your body. They are not just happening arbitrarily to you; you can act with purpose and change the way your body feels right now. Yoga forms offer many opportunities to purposefully create dynamics in your body and to practice feeling them.

## One more way to notice muscle dynamics: Self-touch

Many people who have come through our clinic over the years have found it difficult to feel certain parts of their body and, therefore, muscle dynamics associated with those body parts. In fact, I would say that this is a normal experience in the context of complex trauma. When this is the case, one possibility is to use one's own hands to get a tactile sense of what is happening in a particular muscle. For example, I worked with a client who could not feel his arms. It was an eerie and disturbing experience for him to be looking at his arms but not be able to feel any dynamic changes when we experimented with some yoga forms that engaged these muscles. Even when his arm muscles were intensely engaged in a form like a push-up, he reported that while he could see the muscles in his arms he could not feel them. Operating under the assumption that this was not a neurological condition (a reasonable possibility and one that may need to be looked into for some clients) because he was under the care of a physician and had no indications of such a problem, we proceeded to create an exercise together that we thought might give him a chance to feel his arms (which he was interested in being able to do). We would sit in a chair and flex and extend our arms at the elbow and use our own hands to feel what was happening to the biceps (upper arm muscles in the front of the arm) and the triceps (upper arm muscles in the back of the arm). He and I both noticed we could feel with our hands these muscles change when we moved between bending and straightening. There was something very relieving for this man to be able to use his own hand to feel his arm muscles change like this based on the gestures he was making. (In fact, to reflect back on our discussion above about "purpose," in my observation, it was as if he was moving his arm like this because he wanted to feel his muscle dynamics—he was moving with a purpose). We ended up doing a very detailed investigation over the course of many months and, using a variety of yoga forms, into all of the different things we could feel happening in our arm muscles by using our hands to feel them. Eventually, in this case, he was able to feel his arm muscles without directly using his hands, though we came back to that practice regularly and tried it with different muscles as well.

The invitation is to feel free to experiment with using your own hands in any form as another way to feel muscle dynamics. Facilitators can present this option as another choice for clients and can also feel free to try it themselves if they are interested.

## From estrangement to familiarity

Many traumatized people have the experience of not feeling safe or at home in their bodies. This sense of estrangement often involves not being able to feel certain parts of the body or certain muscular actions but it also relates to some of the theoretical underpinnings to TSY that were discussed in Chapter 1. In this case, complex trauma theory suggests that "for the infant and young child exposed to chaos, violence, or neglect interpretation of sensory stimuli will become infused with danger. At this stage, given non verbal processing, cues for potential danger will generalize and be solidified without language" (Blaustein & Kinniburgh, 2010, p. 14). For our clients, things that happen in their muscles (muscle dynamics), if they are feel-able at all, are often experienced as external sensory stimuli (exteroception): feelings that we perceive as coming at us from the outside. For our clients, a muscle contracting or extending is often interpreted as confusing and dangerous because the connection between the sensation and purposeful action is not clear: I am not making that happen; rather, it is happening to me from the outside. In addition, the feeling can often be generalized so that rather than feeling a specific muscle contract (like a bicep), we just feel a generalized sensation of intensity that we cannot pinpoint in any one part of the body. This experience further exacerbates the alienation from our body and the terror associated with random sensations that are unknowable and uncontrollable.

As an example, I worked with a 16-year-old girl with a history of early life trauma who would, on an almost daily basis, break down wailing and sobbing uncontrollably and hitting her head against a wall and sometimes collapsing into near catatonia often for an hour or two. When she would talk with staff during these episodes, she would say things like "I feel pain in my body but I don't know where it is coming from" or "I can't figure out where this feeling is in my body!" (Again, there did not seem to be a medical basis for these body feelings, though that is certainly a possibility that should be accounted for when working with anybody.) For this girl, the displaced body feeling was part of the experience. Our work together with TSY revolved around trying to find specific things in her body that she could feel. One day, after many months of working together, she felt the muscles in her upper back when we stretched our shoulders back. She could feel the specific action of drawing her shoulder blades closer together and then she noticed she could feel when she reached her arms forward that her shoulder blades separated a little bit. We experimented with this for a few minutes and I asked her if she noticed that she could create these different feelings in her body based on whether she was moving her shoulders forward or back and she said, with a smile, "yes!" She noticed that she was in charge of the feeling in her body based on what she was doing with her shoulders. This was the beginning of her having a new relationship with her body where sensation was not always generalized and terrifying.

## Breathwork as a dynamic process

One of the most dynamic processes that we are all constantly involved with is breathing. As long as we are alive we are breathing. The truth is we are breathing when we are traumatized and we are also breathing after we are traumatized; breath is part of every experience that we have. With TSY we use breath in some specific ways as part of treatment.

In terms of the scholarly literature at this point most of the research associated in some way with breath and trauma involves the PTSD paradigm and conditions called sleep-disordered breathing (Krakow, et al., 2001) and sleep apnea (Sharafkhaneh, et al., 2005). These conditions do involve the actions of breathing and they are very interesting. As research progresses, I suspect they may well eventually have much greater bearing on TSY than is currently the case. However, at this time, there is just not enough information for us to draw any useful conclusions in terms of how we use TSY to treat trauma specifically based on this literature. However, that does not mean that we don't attend to breath very seriously, as we will see.

As we make our way toward some breathing practices, it is

also worth noting that there have been anecdotal stories told and observations made by us and others who treat complex trauma, which seem to suggest a connection between trauma and chronic breath holding or regular breathing in a shallow, choppy, erratic way. I want to be clear that even though I and my colleagues are aware of these anecdotes they have not led us to conclude that there is any one specific, defining breathing pattern attributable to complex trauma. Instead, we are inclined at this point to suspect that, as a result of chronic trauma exposure, no one person's experience with breath is completely transferrable to another. But that is perfectly okay in the context of TSY where the subjective experience trumps the objective every time. The most important thing about breath in the context of TSY is that it is a fundamentally dynamic phenomenon that involves a lot of body movements (rib cage, abdominal muscles, shoulders, and more), which we can interact with.

Because of these dynamics, breath provides many opportunities to feel things in the body. That said, it is clear to us through our experience that breath is also a very complex and fraught phenomenon in the context of trauma. Many of our clients have reported to us how difficult it is just to breathe freely. We hear things like "I wish I could breathe better"; "I want to breathe but my body won't let me"; "I don't take deep breaths because I don't want to be alive"; "I find myself holding my breath, even now, so no one will notice me."

Yoga has a very old and rich history of working with breath, and interested readers will find many resources that discuss detailed and complex breathing practices (for examples, see Farhi, 1996; Feuerstein, 1998). With TSY, we take a very simple approach to breath. For our purposes, we do not use our breath as a way to change our physiology: we don't practice breathing in order to get energized (activate the sympathetic nervous system) or to calm ourselves down (activate the parasympathetic nervous system). We do not approach breath as if there is one way to breathe that is "better" than another. For us, breathing is primarily just another way to experience the dynamic possibilities that having a body entails; to notice what we feel; and to make some choices. Working with the dynamic qualities of breath also offers opportunities for our clients to have *new* body experiences that may be very different from trauma (assuming that trauma limits or constrains our capacity to breathe in some way). Any time we breathe or move in a new way as part of trauma treatment we begin to challenge, in a gentle but clear way, the traumatic notion that my body is not capable of having new experiences and that all it can do is hunker down and resist traumatic memories that are hidden inside every seemingly innocuous muscle movement.

I'd like to share with you some specific practices that provide opportunities for experiencing breath as a dynamic thing. We will focus in detail on a practice called Sun Breaths in Chapter 7 when we explore rhythms so I won't go into it here other than to say that Sun Breaths incorporate the synchronization of breath and movement. In Chapter 7, Sun Breaths will be discussed for their rhythmical quality but it is also possible to emphasize the dynamic qualities of the form instead (i.e., "when you breathe in and reach your arms up you may feel muscles in your back and shoulders strengthening and lengthening"). In addition to Sun Breaths, there are four more breathing practices that we use as part of TSY that I want to emphasize here. Each one of these breathing practices can be incorporated into any yoga form in this book, and each one focuses mostly on the dynamic qualities of breath in some way: *noticing breath, movement of breath, adding a little breath,* and *nasal breath.*

## Noticing breath

One way to experiment with noticing breath is for the TSY facilitator to invite an awareness of breath from time to time throughout the practice by simply stating, "You may notice that you are breathing." This invitatory statement calls attention to breath without imposing any expectations and without requiring any further interaction. It is presented more as a statement of fact than as something that needs to be acted on in some way. For a comment like "you may notice that you are breathing" to be sensible it doesn't matter *how* you are breathing (short choppy breath, long shallow breath, etc.); it is just an invitation to notice that you *are* breathing.

Another way to practice noticing breath is to experiment with feeling some of the physical qualities or sensations related to breath. For example, you may feel the movement of the air around your nose or mouth. This also includes the possibility of feeling some of the ways your body moves when you breathe. For example, your rib cage moves with each breath and this may be feel-able (more specifically, the muscles called intercostals that are between your ribs are active when we breathe and because they are attached to our ribs, our rib cage moves); also, there is movement around our stomach as well as in our chest and upper back. There is one big muscle in particular called the diaphragm, considered to be the primary breathing muscle, that sits more or less around your lower ribs. With each breath you might feel some particular activity around your lower ribs due to this muscle.

All of these things are potentially feel-able and provide ways for us to notice that we are breathing. In this way, breath becomes another thing to interocept. As in any interoceptive practice, we do not require people to feel anything, we just invite them to notice what they feel, even if that is nothing at all in terms of body movement associated with breathing.

A general encouragement to TSY facilitators is that when you introduce breath as a feel-able thing, make sure you yourself can feel the dynamic. In other words, as long as you can feel your rib cage move, then you can feel free to say to your client, "You may notice some movement around your rib cage when you breathe." If you cannot feel your ribs move when you breathe, better to not bring it up. I am encouraging a general authenticity to your use of TSY that begins with the "truth" of your own interoceptive experience. If you don't feel something but bring it up as feel-able, the whole endeavor lacks an integrity that is vital.

## Movement of breath

Along with movement within our body associated with breath, breath itself is also moving. The TSY facilitator can add a simple reminder that "breath is moving" at different points throughout the practice. We can safely say this because it is true. Someone might be breathing very slow, very fast, erratically, shallowly, and so on, but, as long as he or she is alive, there is movement to the breathing patterns. The movement of breath that I am referring to here is a relationship between the inhale and the exhale.

## Adding a little breath

This practice provides an opportunity to use muscles in a new way or new muscles altogether. For example, most of us emphasize some muscles over others when we breathe; we get into a rut. For traumatized people this breathing rut may be related to trauma; for example, we have had people tell us that one way they learned not to be found by a perpetrator was to breathe in a very shallow, quiet way and that this breathing pattern has become habitual. However, for our purposes, whether or not a breathing pattern is directly connected with trauma isn't even the most important thing. The important thing is that by adding a little breath we may give ourselves access to a new dynamic in our body and therefore to something new that is feel-able.

To get this one started the invitation could be something like "beginning from wherever you are, if you like, you could experiment with adding a little to your inhale and a little to your exhale." (In general, we encourage our clients who are interested in adding a little breath to experiment with making their inhale the same as their exhale, especially so that they don't end up overdoing an inhale, which might cause them to feel lightheaded or anxious.) The purpose is primarily to investigate what it feels like in the body to take a slightly deeper breath without any expectations or coercion. You might invite your clients to notice if, when they add a little breath, they feel some ways that their bodies move as they breathe. Your clients, heretofore, may not have felt their bodies move as they breathed and they may only start to feel the dynamic qualities of their breath once they experiment with breathing a little deeper than normal. In this way, adding a little breath provides an opportunity to have a new body experience. In the context of trauma, new body experiences may well elicit traumatic memories but they also give your clients a chance to step out of rigid trauma paradigms and experience a new visceral sense of possibility. My suggestion is that you, as a clinician working within the sphere of your professional training and licensure if appropriate, will know how to help your clients manage this complex experience that new breathing patterns will bring up (in other words, there will be a time to talk about it and a time to experience it).

## Nasal breath

This last one can be introduced simply as a way to try something specific with breath, not as a way to identify nasal breathing as *better* than mouth breathing. The TSY facilitator can say something like "If you like, you can experiment with breathing in and out through your nose." It may be that your client, for whatever reason, has been breathing primarily through his mouth and an invitation to try some nasal breathing might open up possibilities for new experiences. Nasal breathing may activate different muscles. You can invite your client to notice if he feels like he is using different muscles in his body when he breathes through his nose as opposed to his mouth.

When I introduce nasal breathing I always remind my clients that they can always go back to mouth breathing at any time if nasal breathing is uncomfortable.

Again, and this can't be emphasized enough, no one way of breathing is inherently better than another in the context of TSY. These exercises are all just opportunities to interact with your body in some new, intentional ways. Your client is always in control and you are always presenting the material in an invitational and not a prescriptive way.

## Conclusions

For survivors of complex trauma, the most common body experiences are the estrangement of feeling nothing at all or the horror of feeling something happening in the body that they cannot exactly pinpoint and over which they have no control. With the practice of sensing muscle dynamics, including those dynamics involved with breathing, we can begin to investigate both tolerable sensation in the body and our ability to make things happen on purpose in specific muscles. We can use any number of yoga forms and breathing practices but always remember that the forms and breathing practices are just a means to an end, not the ends themselves. The client gets to choose which forms and breathing practices are useful; we only present ideas. Ultimately, the more comfortable we get with having a body that is feel-able and muscle dynamics that are both very specific and under our control, the more we heal the impact of complex trauma.

The final aspect of trauma treatment that we will focus on involves various aspects of the phenomenon of rhythm, including reestablishing a sense of movement and flow right within the context of our body; our perceptions of the passage of time; and connection with others.

# 7

# RHYTHM

THIS CHAPTER OPENS WITH THREE DIFFERENT CASE vignettes that illustrate different aspects of rhythm as applied in trauma-sensitive yoga (TSY).

## Reclaiming movement: A case story

"The first time we tried this I felt like I was being attacked again. Do you remember?" Vital said, while she and her therapist experimented with lifting up and holding their legs.

"As soon as I felt my leg muscles, it was like they were coming up behind me right then." Vital had survived captivity, repeated rape, and torture in the Central African Republic, and she had eventually become a refugee in Europe where she met her therapist, Maria. Vital and Maria had worked together for about 2 years. The Leg Lift was done from a seated posture in a chair (see the Leg Lift exercises in Chapter 8 for examples), and they had started doing this form together, among others, very soon after they met. The first time they tried the Leg Lift together, Maria had simply introduced it as another form they could try. After a few seconds of lifting and extending her leg, Vital became

very upset and tearful and she eventually shut down. They
stopped the TSY session immediately and moved into a
talk-oriented process but Vital was still deeply shaken, even
at the end of the session. They made a plan to check in
by phone the next day and to meet again in 3 days. Vital
couldn't even find the words to explain her experience to
Maria until the next time they met in person. When she was
able to talk about it, Vital said that as soon as she lifted her
leg off the floor she literally felt like her attackers (several
of whom she had known very personally since childhood,
having attended school together side by side for years) were
right behind her in Maria's office about to attack. Vital was
a physically strong and fit person, and she told Maria how,
before all of the horrible things happened to her, she used
to love to run and, particularly, to feel the strength in her
leg muscles. For Vital, running was a way for her to, as she
said, "connect with the body" and "feel alive," and it felt as if
this had been taken from her. She told Maria that she hadn't
been able to run since coming to Europe because, she now
realized, she couldn't stand to feel her leg muscles engage:
"when I'd feel my leg muscles activate, for some reason, I
didn't feel safe." Doing the Leg Lift brought all of this more
immediately to her consciousness for the first time and she
realized how much she missed being able to run. Vital now
experienced this as a profound loss and she became interested in, as she said, "reclaiming" her legs. Vital told Maria,
"I want to feel comfortable running again."

As they talked this over together, they decided to keep
experimenting with the Leg Lift but to modify it so that Vital
could be in control of the experience. They decided to make

it a movement rather than a static hold because Vital noticed, after they tried both options a couple of times, that she felt more comfortable with the movement. They started off by trying three of these leg lift movements with each leg; both Vital and Maria moved at their own pace. Vital noticed that it was critically important that she be in charge of moving her leg at her own pace but that it was also important that Maria was willing to do the leg lifts but not try to control Vital's pace. In other words, what made this work for Vital was that both she and Maria were doing the leg lifts together but that each was responsible for her own pace.

After a few weeks they tried five movements like this with each leg. Within a couple of months they were doing ten leg lifts (Vital decided this would be the maximum) and it was at this point that Vital began to jog again.

## Things begin and end: A case story

Juan spent a large portion of his time in therapy talking about how much he hated his body and how he literally fantasized about not having a body. On a hunch, Juan's therapist told him about TSY and they decided to try a few forms together. One of the forms they tried together was a seated Forward Fold (see Chaper 8 for some variations). Upon trying the form for the first time, Juan realized a conflict playing out within his body in relation to the form: on the one hand he noticed that he actually liked the feeling of the stretch in his back muscles when he folded forward (again, this was unusual and unexpected for Juan because he couldn't remember liking a body feeling before) but at the same time he became terrified every time he would incline forward even a little bit. Juan knew he was terrified because he realized he couldn't breathe, though he didn't have any direct feelings that he would be able to identify as fear and he did not experience any clear memories associated with folding forward. He just noticed he could barely breathe and this really scared him.

With regards to TSY, Juan's therapist focused on two things: the fact that Juan could feel a stretch in his back and that he wanted to have access to this feeling in his body (he liked it) and the issue of breath (for more on breath, see Chapter 6). She did not attempt to investigate any trauma content with Juan related to folding forward and/or not being able to breathe nor did she ask Juan to attempt to make meaning out of his experience. In order to give Juan an opportunity to experience the feeling of muscles stretching in his back (Juan's therapist recognized how rare it was for Juan to have a body feeling that he actually liked), she introduced a practice called the countdown. The countdown is when the TSY facilitator counts down from a given number to zero while a form is held (as always, the student or client can change a form or come out of it at any moment for any reason). The countdown gives an opportunity to experiment with a form for a short, very clearly delineated period of time. The key idea with regards to using the countdown is that everyone knows an end is always in sight and that the current experience will not last forever. After trying several different amounts of time together (a count of two, a count of five, and a count of three), Juan noticed that a count of three was just enough. He could feel his back but he could still breathe (the two count wasn't quite enough for him to feel his back and the five count was too much and he noticed he started to have a hard time breathing). After a few weeks of folding forward for a count of three, Juan noticed that he could breathe fine, knowing there was an end in sight, and also that he could enjoy the feeling of muscles stretching in his back.

## Connection with others: A case story

For Joann, the yoga class was her only social activity. She was the head of a research team at a lab and had many public responsibilities but she considered her "work self" very different from her "other self," the person who had experienced physical and emotional abuse at home as a child and then subsequently within several intimate relationships over the course of her adult life. The yoga class, along with being her only social activity, was also the only thing she did with other people who, she knew, had also experienced trauma, though they never really talked about it. Her favorite part of the class was the Sun Breaths. This was when they would breathe and move together. The instructor would invite students to either match her pace or to go at their own pace. Sometimes Joann would intentionally match the instructor and other times she would experiment with her own rhythm. While she really appreciated having the options, there was one time when she noticed that everyone, including herself, was going at the same pace and she experienced a feeling of safety and connection to the people around her that she had never felt before.

# Three different aspects of rhythm

Three different aspects of rhythm apply to the practice of TSY, which we will explore in this chapter: (1) immobilization versus movement, (2) passage of time, and (3) isolation versus connection with others. In our examples above we can see all three at work in different ways. Let's take a look at each aspect of rhythm in some more detail.

## Immobilization versus movement

Let's begin with a clinical term that is associated with post-traumatic stress disorder (PTSD): avoidance. This is a behavioral symptom that must be present in order for someone to be diagnosed with PTSD and it involves a person staying away from people or places that remind them, either explicitly or implicitly, of their traumatic experiences. In the case of avoidance, what is most pertinent is that our body experience of the phenomenon involves things we cannot do, movements we cannot make, places we cannot go. It is this restriction on what we can and cannot do with our bodies as a result of trauma that opens the door for using rhythm as part of trauma treatment.

Judith Herman used the term "constriction" as a nuanced variation of avoidance, which she described as "avoiding any situation reminiscent of the past trauma, or any initiative that might involve future planning and risk" (1992, p. 47). The key word here is "initiative." This is an action word that implies doing something with your body, and Herman suggests that her iteration of complex PTSD involves avoiding some instances of initiative as a direct impact of trauma exposure. Similarly, Bessel van der Kolk observes that one way to conceptualize trauma is as a failure of the organism to mount a successful defense against a threat, which then becomes a "conditioned behavioral response" that he calls "immobilization" (van der Kolk, 2006, p. 7). Again, the language here is very purposeful and not incidental; the overarching experience of a person who is traumatized is a physical one of chronic constriction and immobilization; it is experienced in the body, not in the mind. Avoidance, constriction, and immobilization are the antithesis of movement, the antithesis of rhythm. Constriction and immobilization short-circuit the natural movement inherent in the organism and calcify our physical experience into more or less one rigid thing, which is to use the body to avoid traumatic memory.

If we accept this characterization then we have to think about how we can address it. How do we treat an inability to move? (And, again, I am not pathologizing this experience but rather suggesting it is an understandable consequence of complex trauma; who among us would willingly expose ourselves to hellishly painful abuse and neglect or any situations that remind us of these experiences?) How do we become unconstricted and mobilized in the face of very real traumatic experiences that are constantly playing out within our bodies? By this point in the book it will come as no surprise to readers that the answer to these questions involves one more step beyond thinking or talking about it, which has been the traditional role of psychotherapy; it is about moving our bodies right now (as we shall see, sometimes in a very purposeful and self-directed way, at other times just for the sake of movement).

Consider the example of Vital above. There was a moment in the process when Vital verbalized her experience with the Leg Lift and then she and her therapist talked together about how they might approach her desire to reclaim her leg muscles. So while talking did play an important part in this case in terms of helping them plan what to do, the treatment actually centered on moving the body, on doing the Leg Lift together, and on Vital being able to control the pace of the movement for herself. Again, some clients may find it very helpful to engage in more of an objective analysis of their experience but some may not and, especially given what we have learned from the neuroscience research, some may not be able to put into words what it feels like to be constricted or immobilized (see van der Kolk, 1994, for a reminder of the impact of trauma on parts of the brain related to speech).

While Vital found it useful and was able to draw a connection between her present experience of feeling overwhelmed by lifting her leg and her past experience of trauma, a more common scenario in our experience would be that someone feels terrified by lifting his leg but doesn't know why. He just has a visceral reaction and that's all there is to it. It may well be that by lifting his leg he has suddenly been exposed to an implicit reminder of trauma. He may have unconsciously been avoiding this action of lifting his leg because the motoric activity itself may contain traumatic memories. This highlights for us the importance within TSY of never forcing experiences on people, being attuned to when our client finds something like a leg lift intolerable in the moment, and knowing that we can always move out of a form and/or into another form. However, if the form is tolerable you can invite your client to notice it for what it is: in the case of the leg lift, activity in the leg muscles. In Vital's case, she noticed she had been unable to move her legs in any way that caused her muscles to engage to a certain degree where they were feel-able. Moving her leg into the Leg Lift caused enough muscular activity for her to experience what is commonly referred to as a triggered reaction and she became very upset. The work between her and her therapist was to find a way for her to move her leg in a very controlled fashion, to thereby reclaim movement in her legs, and to eventually run again.

The key to using TSY to practice movement is to accept that physical movement alone, without the intellectual association with trauma, may be enough to allow people to have new, healing experiences (again, granted, some of your clients will also benefit greatly from being able to talk to you about their experiences, including associating particular movements with trauma).

## Passage of time

Another important aspect of rhythm is time, namely the experience that things begin and end. While this is a topic that can quickly pull me outside of my area of expertise, I think there is some relevant clinical material that needs to be cited regarding trauma and time. Another way we can objectively judge an organism's relationship to time, and particularly to the passage of time, is related to sleep patterns. A healthy organism operates with a highly attuned internal clock. The literature indicates that the parts of the brain most involved in our sleep and wakefulness patterns (as well as other important rhythmical patterns like eating and sex) are the thalamus and the hypothalamus (Saper, Scammell, & Lu, 2005). These brain regions are associated with the interoceptive pathways, which we know are compromised by trauma (see Chapters 1 and 2 for more about the interoceptive pathways). We also know from the research that traumatized people are more likely to experience sleep disturbances than their nontraumatized counterparts (Chapman et al., 2011). These findings point to a disturbance in fundamental circadian rhythms, our basic sense of time on an organism level, as a result of trauma.

Another aspect of time that seems to be impacted by trauma comes more from an anecdotal perspective based on what clients tell therapists (and occasionally yoga teachers), which is that bad things, even difficult things, don't feel like they are going to end. In particular, I invite readers to consider the experience that has been discussed previously in this book that has direct bearing, which is that traumatized people are in a sense compelled to orbit around their trauma ad infinitum. That is, the trauma is so compelling on an interpersonal and neurobiological level that it never ends; it's like having the same song stuck on replay. With TSY we want to give our clients the possibility to press "stop" and to play another song if they choose. Another way to formulate this phenomenon is that, for traumatized people, time stops moving; things stop beginning and ending.

Consider again the Vital example. It turned out that time had stopped moving for her in a very real way though she didn't know it until she was invited to try the Leg Lift. She hadn't realized that beginnings and endings had been replaced by trauma until she lifted her leg and contracted the large muscles on top of her thigh, and, instead of feeling her quadriceps contract, she felt like she was about to be attacked. This kind of experience is very common for clients at the Trauma Center. In a very real way, time had become calcified for Vital in her leg muscles. They were no longer her muscles that could move through time, contracting and extending and resting; they were where trauma was experienced by her as a constant presence in her body. While Vital was able to notice that her leg muscles had in effect been hijacked by trauma, most of our clients at the Trauma Center who have survived early childhood trauma cannot make that connection between an experience in their bodies and the abuse and neglect they endured as infants. That's okay. In fact, TSY in no way requires this cognitive connection in order to be a successful treatment. The process would be to just work with each of your clients to find parts of the body that are feel-able for them and begin to experiment with noticing things happening, sensations changing, in those muscles based on the forms they are doing. If one body part causes too much distress, just move on to another body part. The purpose of this work is to be able to use your body to feel things begin (like a muscle contract) and to feel things end (when you make that muscle stop contracting). The work is *not* to expose people to parts of their body that cause them distress as a way to reframe their relationship with that particular body part. Any part of the body will do for this kind of TSY practice.

Further, as in the Juan example, the facilitator has a key tool available to help her clients reestablish a sense of beginning and ending: we call it the countdown. I use the countdown most often when someone is experimenting with holding a form that is challenging in some way. The challenge could be something physical like using a large muscle group or it could be something more psychological, as in Juan's case. By counting down from five to one or from three to one, you can put an explicit marker on time: this thing we are doing together has begun and it will end when I get to one (of course, we can remind people they are welcome to come out of any form at any time for any reason). While they are in no way obligated to hold the form for your countdown, they have the option and they can rely on the "clock" you are keeping as a way to practice experiencing something intense in their bodies.

Finally, as part of this process, it may be important for the facilitator to give the invitation at the end of the countdown for the client to notice that whatever dynamic he had created in his body is now over and he may feel that change. Your client may try to distinguish a body feeling like a muscle contracting from displaced trauma; giving him a chance to notice what it feels like when that muscle stops contracting both puts an end to the period of time in which the contraction was occurring but it also gives him a chance to feel directly that challenging things do in fact end.

This brings up one final aspect of time: if we have a beginning and an end we also have a middle. The middle is when we are taking the action that was initiated at the beginning (in Juan's case it started with him folding forward). The middle is also when the dynamic we created at the beginning is happening (in Juan's case this was when his back muscles were lengthening) though, in TSY, we may or may not feel these dynamics. Figure 7.1 depicts Juan's experience in relation to time.

**Figure 7.1.** Juan's experience in relation to time.

| Fold forward | holding for countdown | sitting back up straight |
|:---:|:---:|:---:|
| **Beginning** | **Middle** | **End** |

Each yoga form has a beginning, middle, and end. For many clients it will be important for us to help them start to feel this aspect of time right in their bodies.

## Isolation versus connection

Judith Herman has written that "helplessness and isolation are the core experiences of psychological trauma. Empowerment and reconnection are the core experiences of recovery" (1992, p. 197). While I have mentioned her formulation of empowerment as part of trauma treatment throughout this book, in this section I want to focus on isolation versus reconnection. This paradigm suggests that trauma has a tendency to isolate us from others whether it is very explicit, as in being kept captive by a perpetrator, or more implicit, as in feeling like no one understands the things you have been through. In either case, part of treatment involves finding a way back into the company of others. With TSY, we focus on a physical aspect of sharing space with other people, namely, doing things together. As I have noted previously, most clients at the Trauma Center have experienced interpersonal trauma, abuse, or neglect perpetrated by one person on another. Trauma treatment, whether it is individual psychotherapy of any type or a body-based praxis, is also fundamentally a relational thing, something that occurs between people (setting aside such experimental interventions as those being undertaken by the military to use videogame-type interfaces as part of an exposure treatment for combat soldiers with PTSD). If we are to offer good therapies we need to return again and again, in both our understanding and our therapeutic offering, to the relational dynamics of both trauma and treatment. The experience of moving together with another person is an explicit way that we can practice truly being together—sharing space. It is also another aspect of rhythm.

In the Joann example, we have a situation where the rhythmical practice of doing something together is in itself therapeutic. While trauma is something that people do together, it is not truly rhythmical; the power dynamic is so distorted and abusive that it becomes one person doing something *to* someone else. It is not a mutual process where both people have an equal capacity to affect the outcome. Trauma is when one person exerts all of the control and under these conditions a truly rhythmical interaction is not possible. In contrast, an interaction can be considered rhythmical if both parties enter into it through their own choice. A rhythmical interaction is one that is cocreated and where both (or all) parties have equal influence on the outcome. TSY seeks to give clients a chance to have rhythmical interactions as a way to practice reconnection. Because of the interoceptive, invitational, and choice-oriented approach to TSY, the facilitator does not have more power in the relationship than the client. Let's not fool ourselves here: your client comes to you for help and she needs your expertise. I am not suggesting that you withhold or deny that. What I am suggesting is that, with TSY, sharing your expertise does not involve setting yourself up in a position of power over your client but rather involves you attending to your own interoceptive and choice-oriented investigation of the form at hand so that your client is free to do the same. The process becomes another aspect of the shared authentic experience that we previously discussed where both parties have equal power. The relationship, for that moment, is neither hierarchized (i.e., therapist/client or healthy person/unhealthy person, even not traumatized/traumatized) nor externalized where one person must conform to the other. Rather, everyone's attention is internalized and focused on what he or she feels and notices and in this subjective domain there can be no external expert. When the therapist and client do these exercises together they engage in interacting with the same material at the same time and in the same space. There may be what looks like two people moving and breathing at the same time but fundamentally, beneath the surface, there are two people each relating to their own subjective and equally valid experiences and neither actor is imposing his or her experience on the other. I would suggest that when these conditions are met then you are doing trauma treatment in the best sense; you are having a truly rhythmical interaction.

## Sun Breaths

Figure 7.2 and 7.3 offer an example of the movement exercise depicted in the Joann case that invites you and your client to connect on a visceral/somatic level.

These forms are presented as a sequence that involves coordinating movement and breath. Readers may wish to experiment with the Sun Breaths alone or with someone else. In either case, if you like, begin in a comfortable seated form. You may wish to bring your hands to the tops of your legs. As you breathe in, you may wish to experiment with lifting your hands a few inches up from your legs, as depicted in Figure 7.2. As you breathe out, you may wish to bring your hands back down to the tops of your legs. Figure 7.3 shows an option where, on the in breath, you lift your arms higher and this is also a possibility. Feel free to experiment a little

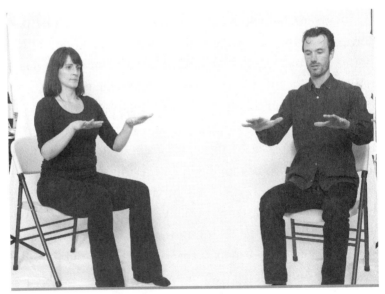

**Figure 7.2.** Sun Breath Variation.

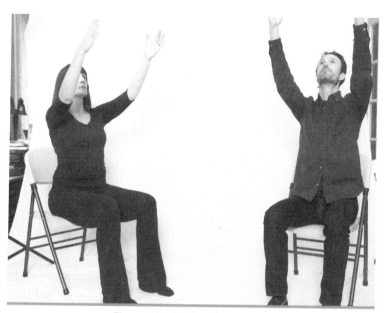

**Figure 7.3.** Sun Breath Variation.

bit with this breathing and moving pattern and with finding a gesture that is relatively comfortable for you. Once you get comfortable enough with the movement pattern, you may wish to find a pace that feels good to you. If you are doing this with someone else, it is okay if both participants go at a different pace. In any case, if you like, give yourself a minute or two to move and breathe at your own pace. The other option, if you are with another person (or more than one), as depicted in the Joann case, is that one of you can set a pace and you can invite the other to experiment with following your pace. The encouragement is to set a pace that feels authentic, comfortable, and natural to you, based on your own interoceptive experience with the form. Finally, you can trade off who sets the pace and who follows if you like.

## Rhythmical attunement in TSY

In the clinical literature when attunement is discussed it is most often of the type described by Daniel Stern as "affect attunement." When Stern writes, in the case of affect attunement, "what is being matched is not the other person's behavior per se but rather, it seems, some aspect of an internal feeling state" (1985, p.142) he indicates that his conceptualization of attunement seems to focus on an emotional resonance of internal states—happy, sad, hopeful, and so on—that are first experienced by one person and then essentially mirrored by the other. In fact, a good portion of Stern's excellent book *The Interpersonal World of the Infant* is devoted to wondering how one can most effectively attune one's affect so that the other can really sense this connection. While Stern's work focused mostly on the mother-infant dyad, the investigation of affect attunement has broadened to include other relationships and other life stages (Hrynchak & Fouts, 1998). Simply put, with affect attunement the emphasis is on emotional states.

With the kind of attunement we explore in TSY, the emphasis is on the body experience. What happens is that the facilitator and client both become involved in the practice of doing something together, each in charge of his or her own body but at the same time and in the same space. It may be that they have the same interoceptive experience but it is also very likely that they each feel something different. The act of doing something together is itself a kind of attunement that we can call *rhythmical attunement*. This rhythmical attunement then makes other kinds of experiences available, which are themselves other types of attunement, such as the shared processes of interocepting, choosing what to do, and taking action. Once this sort of relationship is established, then both you and your client are free to have your own experiences without imposing them on each other. In one instance your client may say she feels something or tells you she is making a choice to modify a form so that it feels better and you can simply reflect that back: "that's amazing that you felt that" or "that's fantastic that you made a choice to change that stretch so that it felt more comfortable." In another instance one party may feel something and tell the other about it and the other party may then notice a similar feeling in his own body. I personally have had many experiences like this. On one occasion a student and I were experimenting with a seated twist and I focused on the feeling in the muscles around my rib cage. The student said, "I notice some feeling in my hip muscles" and as soon as she said that I also noticed a feeling in my hip muscles! I told her about this experience because it was genuine and it seemed interesting and I felt like that was an aspect of the kind of attunement that TSY makes available.

Finally, another way to consider attunement in this context is that when your client moves to adjust a form, you may follow him with your body or vice versa. Let's imagine that you are practicing raising your arms to shoulder height and taking a few breaths and noticing how that feels. Your client may instead reach his arms up overhead and say, "My neck was getting sore and this feels a lot better." Along with reflecting back how great that noticing and choice making was, you may also raise your arms higher as well. Now you are matching his body movement. You may need to ask "Is it ok with you if I try that as well?" because some people may feel uncomfortable with you matching them like this. Assuming it's ok and you raise your arms, then you notice how that feels for you and possibly you can also feel some kind of dynamic shift around your neck muscles (maybe not and that's ok too—be honest!) Now you are dancing together; you are moving together; you are practicing levels of attunement based on your body experiences.

## Conclusions

Rhythm is an important part of good trauma treatment in general but is a core essential element of TSY. By being attuned to our rhythmical interactions we get to practice finding ways of moving and breathing that are authentically comfortable. By attending to aspects of rhythm we get to have experiences where one person does not impose his or her will on the other but rather, by being committed to the interoceptive process, actually validates the authenticity of the other's felt experience. The countdown technique, an aspect of rhythm, gives us a way to practice noticing when things, particularly challenging things, begin and end.

For, ultimately, healing trauma is about learning viscerally something that is completely shrouded from awareness when one is in trauma's thrall: things end. Once we know in our body that things end then the next part of our life can begin.

# 8

# A PORTFOLIO OF
# YOGA PRACTICES

IN ORDER TO PRACTICE THE CENTRAL CONCEPTS OF TRAUMA-
sensitive yoga (TSY)—interoception, choice making, action
taking, being present, muscle dynamics, and rhythms—you
need yoga forms in which to contextualize them. Along with
the examples I have given throughout the book, in this chapter I present a selection of yoga forms that we use regularly
in our work at the Trauma Center. One thing that readers
will notice is that, because TSY is not intended to target specific symptoms, I will not identify particular forms with particular therapeutic goals. Instead, in keeping with the spirit
of this book, I invite you to think about the entire project of
trauma treatment, at least when it comes to TSY, as giving
your client an opportunity to notice a feeling in her body and
then be able to interact with what she feels in various self-
directed ways. If you like, this is the one and only therapeutic goal regarding TSY. That said, you may need to customize
treatment plans and/or categorize for billing purposes, but I
will leave those details up to each individual and ask you to
use your best clinical judgment.

For ease of access and consistency, all of these forms are

chair based. They are not meant to represent an exhaustive list but are merely a sample. That said, there is enough material here for years of TSY practice mostly because repetition is not anathema in TSY. In fact, repeating a form does not mean that the experience is always the same (remember Heraclitus and his river?). That is, a person may have an entirely new experience with the same form each time he or she experiments with it. As I have noted before, the forms are just a means to an end and the end is to have body experiences that are feel-able and with which your clients can effectively interact. In this regard some, indeed most, of your clients may find it very helpful to repeat the same forms over and again. Please do not be afraid to repeat the same forms, especially if that is what a client wants to do.

No special training beyond this book is required in order to be able to use these practices, though the encouragement is to not force anything and only do what is comfortable for you and your client. The formatting for this chapter is intended to make it easy for readers to photocopy pages of interest in order to customize a yoga practice. Although the forms are laid out in a linear fashion there is no one way to approach them. You can start with any form that you like and end whenever you want. Some people may want to pick one form to focus on; others may want several.

Most important, along with the pictures, this chapter will give you enough language to create the physical part of the form (this will be indicated by the subheading "Suggested Anatomical Language") and each form will spotlight one theme from the book as a place to begin and some language that you can use to present that theme through the form (this will be indicated by the subheading "TSY Theme Spotlight"). The anatomical language I provide can be used verbatim but it could also be used as a guide to help you develop your own language. The encouragement is to use a minimal amount of anatomical language, just enough for your client to successfully orient to the form, so you can spend most of your time on the TSY content (the material outlined in Chapters 2–7).

Once you create the physical structure of the form, you can start with the information on the TSY theme spotlight. However, just because I spotlight one theme per form doesn't mean that you or your client may not want to use a given form to highlight a different theme or several themes. For example, I've chosen to highlight interoception when I present the Seated Mountain Form, but it could just as easily highlight other aspects of TSY, such as being present. Again, as you get comfortable with the material please feel free to use any form in this book to emphasize any TSY theme that you or your client chooses.

The forms are just static pictures. They come to life through your presentation and through your and your clients' interactions with them.

The suggestion is that readers continuously review and become comfortable not only with the forms as presented here but also with the content of the previous chapters, which detail the context underlying the presentation of the forms that make TSY a treatment for complex trauma. Without the information provided in Chapters 1 through 7, yoga can very easily become yet another command-oriented, perfection-focused, judgment-inducing process that will in the best case get you nowhere and in the worst case create conditions that will exacerbate trauma symptoms. The guidelines to the forms presented in this chapter and thrughout the book will help you avoid these pitfalls.

**IMPORTANT NOTE:** *Though I present the forms in a particular way, you may work with clients who have major physical injuries or are taking medications that require certain modifications. For example, through the Trauma Center we have worked with war veterans with various amputations and with people on strong medications that make it difficult to stay awake. Though it is beyond the scope of this book to go into such details, every form presented can be modified in some way to suit any body. Please use common sense when considering what forms to experiment with and what language to use to introduce them. For example, if someone is in a hospital bed then you would start from a prone position rather than the seated position that all of the pictures start from. The entire series of forms could be done from a prone position and figuring out how to do that could be an interesting process of discovery and empowerment for therapists and clients. Anyone who uses TSY is engaged in a process of discovering his or her own body— what it feels like, what it can do. The key is for therapist and client to find what variation of a form is accessible to them and to start from there. Finally, as with any physical activity, if your client has a particular health condition that is of concern, he or she should check with a doctor before proceeding.*

## Seated Mountain Form

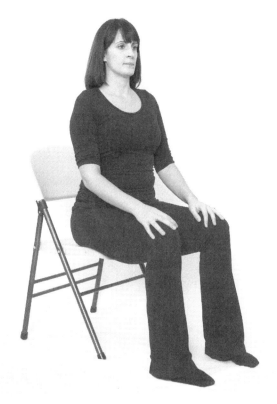

**Suggested anatomical language:** If you like, you may wish to experiment with sitting up comfortably tall in your chair. Maybe you could bring your feet to the floor at about hips' distance apart with your ankles under your knees. Perhaps lengthen slightly up through the top of your head.

**TSY theme spotlight**: *Interoception*: You may feel your body lengthening up.

## Lateral Neck Stretch

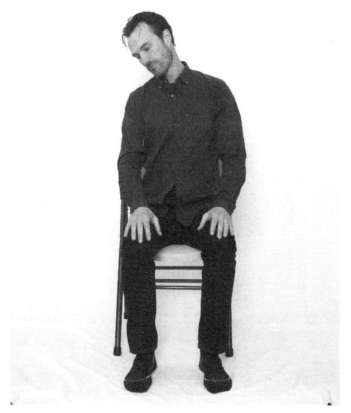

**Suggested anatomical language**: A lateral movement is a movement to the side. If you like, you could gently tilt your head to one side. When you tilt to one side, the muscles on one side of your neck will lengthen. Maybe after a few breaths on one side, you could tilt to the other side for a few breaths.

**TSY theme spotlight**: *Interoception*: When you tilt to one side, you may notice a feeling in the side of your neck that is lengthening.

## Shoulder Circles

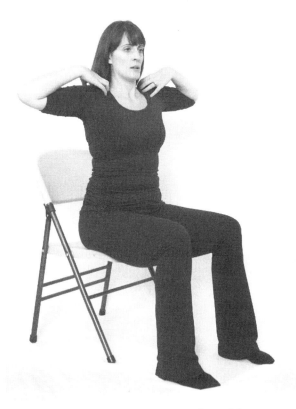

**Suggested anatomical language**: If you like, you could bring your fingertips to the tops of your shoulders and experiment with making circles with your elbows.

**TSY theme spotlight**: *Choice making*: Notice that you can make the circles in either direction. You have a choice. You can move continuously in one direction or you can switch direction a couple of times.

## Gentle Spinal Twist

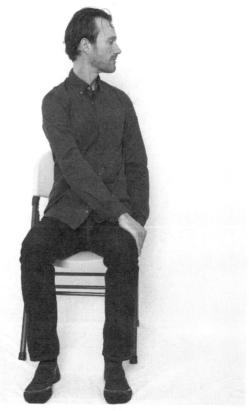

**Suggested anatomical language**: If you like, feel free to experiment with turning to one side. The encouragement is to stay as comfortably tall as you can; in other words, keep your spine comfortably tall. Feel free to place your hands anywhere that is comfortable for you. After a few breaths on one side, you may wish to turn to the other side.

**TSY theme spotlight**: *Choice making*: Notice that you are in charge of how much you turn. You may choose to turn just a little bit or to make the twist a little bit more pronounced. How much you choose to turn is up to you.

## Back and Shoulder Stretch, Variation 1

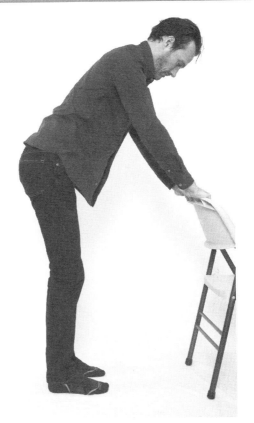

**Suggested anatomical language**: If you like, and if the space you have available allows, you may wish to stand at the back of your chair. Placing your hands on the back of the chair, you may wish to take a step or two back.

**TSY theme spotlight**: *Taking action*: When you stand up, you may notice some muscles that you use to help you stand. If you like, you can experiment with moving from sitting to standing a few times and noticing any muscles that you feel in your body that help you stand.

## Back and Shoulder Stretch, Variation 2

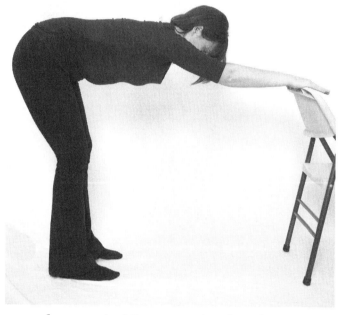

**Suggested anatomical language**: Another choice might be to take several steps back. Feel free to give yourself a moment to breathe in whatever variation of this form that you choose. **TSY theme spotlight**: *Muscle dynamics*: You might notice some feeling in your back or shoulders.

## Hip Stretch 1

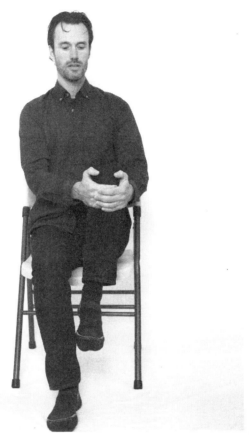

**Suggested anatomical language**: If you like, from the Seated Mountain Form, reach down and gently draw one knee in toward your body. How much you draw your knee in is totally up to you. In this form you may begin to stretch some muscles around your hips. Feel free to take a few breaths and then try the other leg if you like.

**TSY theme spotlight**: *Muscle dynamics*: When you gently draw your knee in, you may notice a feeling around your outer hip. This form tends to stretch outer hip muscles a little bit and you may notice a feeling related to those outer hip muscles stretching.

## Hip Stretch 2, Variation 1

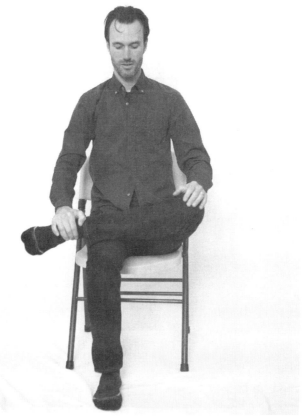

**Suggested anatomical language**: If you like, you could bend one leg and bring that leg on top of the other.

## Hip Stretch 2, Variation 2

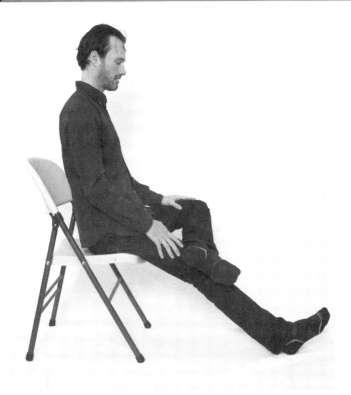

**Suggested anatomical language**: You may wish to straighten that bottom leg. If so, the encouragement is to keep your bottom knee slightly bent so not too much pressure goes into the knee.

## Hip Stretch 2, Variation 3

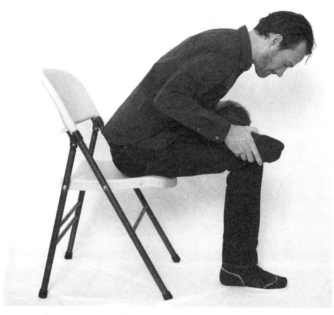

**Suggested anatomical language**: Another possibility is to fold forward.

## Hip Stretch 2, Variation 4

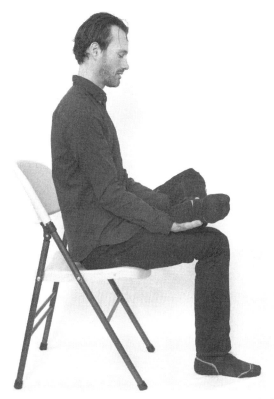

**Suggested anatomical language**: Another possibility is to reach down and gently lift your top leg.

## Gentle Spine Movement

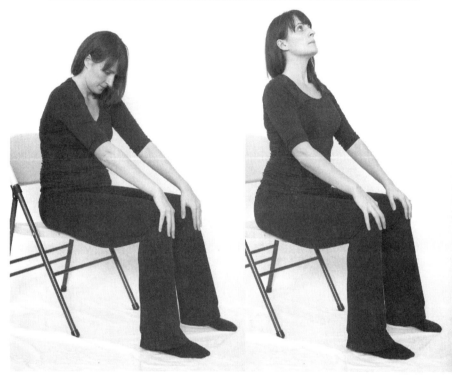

**Suggested anatomical language**: This one could be approached as a movement. If you like, you could gently hold your kneecaps with your hands and curl your upper body slightly forward. The technical term for this gesture is flexing your spine. Another way to say it is rounding your back gently. The second part of the movement is to lift up your chin and sternum toward the sky. This is called extending your spine. If you like, you can oscillate between flexing and extending your spine a few times.

**TSY theme spotlight**: *Rhythm (intrapersonal)*: If you choose to approach this form as a movement, notice that you can control your own pace. You can make the pace faster or slower as you like. If you want, maybe experiment with finding a pace that feels natural to you.

## Shoulder Stretch 1

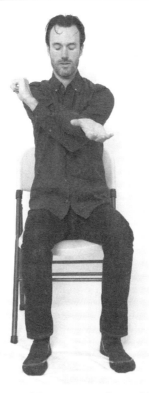

**Suggested anatomical language**: If you like, from the Seated Mountain Form, you could hook one arm under the other. This may stretch some muscles in the back of your shoulder, around your shoulder blade. Feel free to try both sides if you like.

**TSY theme spotlight**: *Interoception*: You may notice a feeling around or between your shoulder blades.

## Shoulder Stretch 2

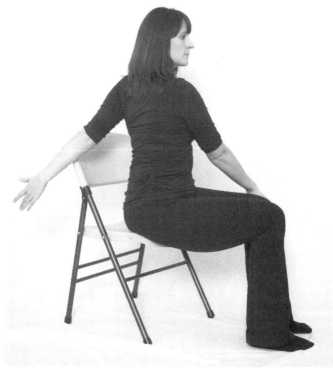

**Suggested anatomical language**: This form stretches the opposite muscles of Shoulder Stretch 1 (though you certainly do not have to do them together). If you like, from the Seated Mountain Form, rotate your entire body about 45 degrees in one direction. Then, if you rotated to your left, you could reach your left arm back around to the right side of the chair. This stretches some muscles in the front of your shoulder. Feel free to take a few breaths and then switch sides if you like.

**TSY theme spotlight**: *Interoception*: You may notice a feeling in the front of your shoulder.

## Leg Lift, Variation 1

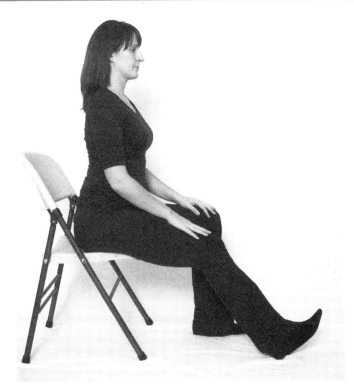

**Suggested anatomical language**: If you like, from the Seated Mountain Form, you could experiment with straightening and then lifting one leg off the ground. This causes some leg muscles to engage.

**TSY theme spotlight**: *Muscle dynamics*: You may notice some feeling in the top of your leg.

## Leg Lift, Variation 2

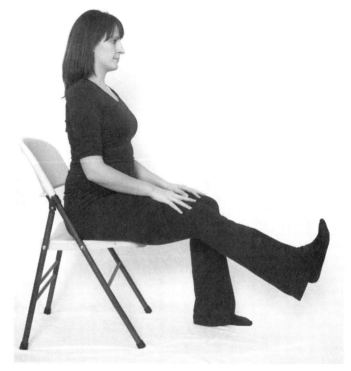

**Suggested anatomical language**: You could lift your leg a bit more.

**TSY theme spotlight**: *Muscle dynamics*: In either variation of this form you may notice the muscles in the top of your leg (called quadriceps) become more engaged when you lift your leg. You may feel these muscles become more engaged or, if you like, you could place one hand on the top of your thigh as another way to feel what happens to those muscles when they become engaged.

## Forward Fold, Variation 1

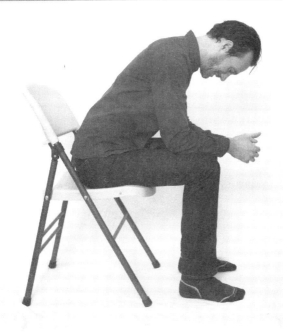

**Suggested anatomical language**: If you like, from the Seated Mountain Form, you may wish to lean forward.

**TSY theme spotlight**: *Choice making*: You have several variations with this forward fold. You can choose any of the three variations presented. If you like, you could try each variation, notice how it feels in your body, and then let that help you choose which one to do. Feel free to give yourself a moment in whichever variation you choose. Another thing to notice about choice is that you are never stuck with one. Just because you choose one variation doesn't mean you can't change your mind at some point. You always have the control to change the variation of the form or to come out of it at any point.

## Forward Fold, Variation 2

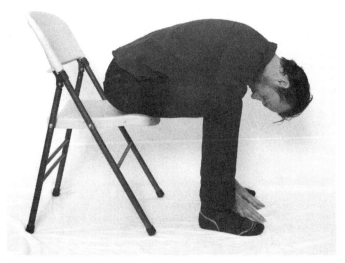

**Suggested anatomical language**: Another option is to toe-heel your feet a little wider than your hips and fold forward so your fingertips touch the floor (you could also place your hands on something like a pillow or a yoga block if you have one).

## Forward Fold, Variation 3

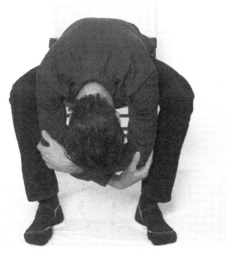

**Suggested anatomical language**: Another option is to bring your opposite hand to your opposite elbow and hang freely forward.

## Seated Warrior, Variation 1

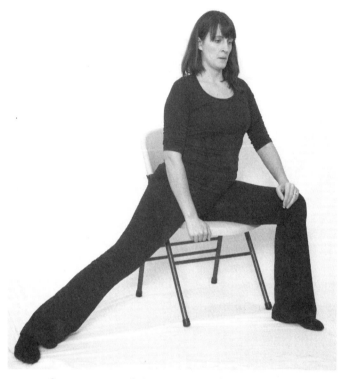

**Suggested anatomical language**: If you like, you could extend one leg to the side.

**TSY theme spotlight**: *Muscle dynamics:* When you extend your leg, the muscles lengthen. You may notice a feeling related to the muscles lengthening in your leg.

## Seated Warrior, Variation 2

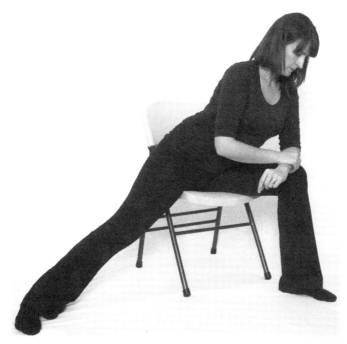

**Suggested anatomical language**: Another option is to lean into your leg that is still bent.

**TSY theme spotlight**: *Present moment:* When you lean into your leg like this, you may feel the pressure that is created on the top of your leg as you gently press your weight through your arm. This contact is something you might feel as sensation.

## Seated Warrior, Variation 3

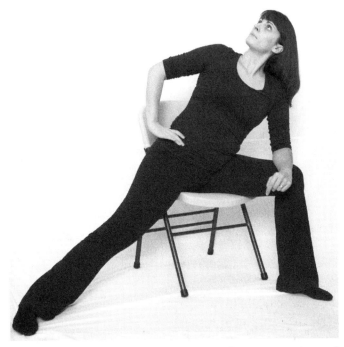

**Suggested anatomical language**: Another option is to place one hand on your hip and gently roll that shoulder open. You may wish to look up or you could look down.

**TSY Theme Spotlight:** *Choice making*: Notice when you can look up or down (or anywhere in between). Maybe one way of rotating your neck feels better than the other options. That's one way to help you make a choice: what feels better.

## Seated Warrior, Variation 4

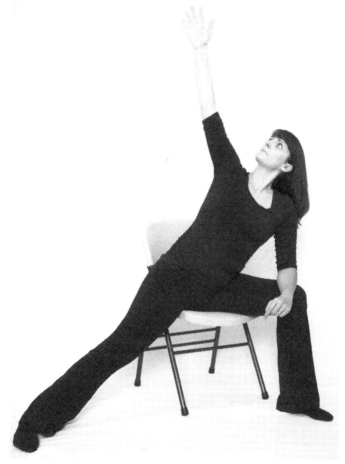

**Suggested anatomical language**: Another option is to extend your top arm toward the sky. Feel free to experiment with this option and then, if you like, switch sides.

## Sun Breath, Variation 1

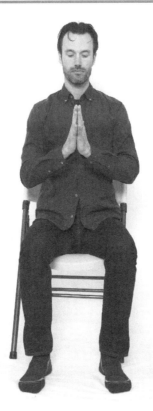

Chapter 6 contained a variation of the Sun Breath exercises that invited a practice of breathing and moving in a synchronized way. Other variations of that exercise follow.

**Suggested anatomical language**: If you like, you can begin with your palms together and then, on an inhale, you could expand your arms to your sides. With the exhale, you may want to bring your palms back together. Feel free to experiment with this gesture a few times if you like.

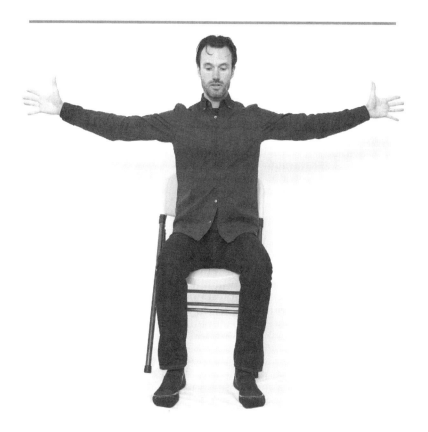

**TSY theme spotlight**: *Rhythm (interpersonal)*: If you like, you could experiment with matching my pace. (There is also the possibility of your client setting the pace and you following him or her.)

## Sun Breath, Variation 2

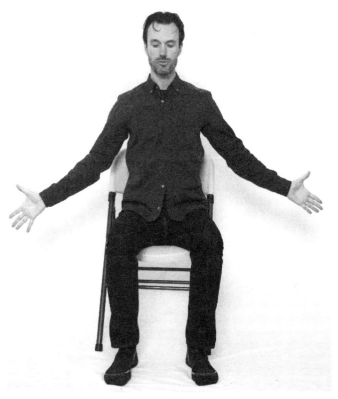

**Suggested anatomical language**: Another possibility for Sun Breaths is to bring your arms to your sides and then, on an inhale, sweep your arms up in a big circle. With the exhale, you could sweep your arms back down to your sides. How high you lift your arms and whether or not you lift your chin when you sweep your arms up is totally up to you. Feel free to experiment with this breathing and moving exercise a few times if you like.

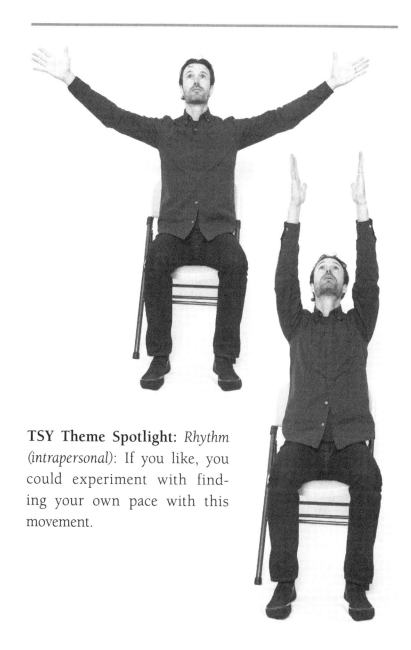

**TSY Theme Spotlight:** *Rhythm (intrapersonal):* If you like, you could experiment with finding your own pace with this movement.

## Rest

*There is no picture for this one
because the invitation is to
find a form that is restful for you.
It could be sitting, standing, or laying down.*

**Suggested anatomical language**: If you like, pause for a moment wherever you are right now or choose any form that is restful for you and come into that form.

**TSY theme spotlight**: *Muscle dynamics*: You may wish to experiment with feeling one muscle that you don't need to use right now. If you are not talking or not chewing something, you may be able to allow your jaw to rest. Maybe you don't need to use some of your leg muscles or arm muscles right now. If you like, pause for a moment and notice if you feel one muscle (or one part of your body) that you purposefully do not need to use in this moment. You might notice what it feels like to not use a muscle. That is the kind of resting dynamic that we practice feeling in TSY.

# REFERENCES

Ainsworth, M. (1979). Infant-mother attachment. *American Psychologist*, 34(10), 932–937.

Anda, R. F., et al. (2009). The relationship of adverse childhood experiences to a history of premature death of family members. *BMC Public Health*, 9(106).

Andreasen, N. (2010). Posttraumatic stress disorder: A history and a critique. *Annals of the New York Academy of Sciences*, 1208, 67–71.

Becker-Weidman, A. (2006). Treatment for children with trauma-attachment disorders: Dyadic developmental psychotherapy. *Child and Adolescent Social Work Journal*, 23, 147–171.

Blaustein, M., & Kinniburgh, K. (2010). *Treating traumatic stress in children and adolescents: How to foster resilience through attachment, self-regulation, and competency.* New York, NY: Guilford Press.

Bossini, L., Tavanti, M., Calossi, S., et al. (2008). Magnetic resonance imaging volumes of the hippocampus in drug-naive patients with post-traumatic stress disorder without comorbidity conditions. *Journal of Psychiatric Research*, 42(9), 752–762.

Bridge, D., & Paller, K. (2012). Neural correlates of reactivation and retrieval-induced distortion. *Journal of Neuroscience*, 32(35), 12,144–12,151.

Chapman, D., et al. (2011). Adverse childhood experiences and sleep disturbances in adults. *Sleep Medicine*, 12(8), 773–779.

Cook, A., Spinazzola, J., et al. (2005). Complex trauma in children and adolescents. *Psychiatric Annals*, 35(5), 390–398.

Corso, P. S., Edwards, V. J., Fang, X., & Mercy, J. A. (2008). Health-related quality of life among adults who experienced maltreatment during childhood. *American Journal of Public Health*, 98(6), 1094–1100.

Coulter, H. D. (2001). *Anatomy of hatha yoga.* Honesdale, PA: Body and Breath.

Courtois, C. (1999). *Recollections of sexual abuse: Treatment principles and guidelines*. New York: W.W. Norton & Co.

Courtois, C., & Ford, J. (2012). *Treatment of complex trauma: A sequenced, relationship-based approach*. New York, NY: Guilford Press.

Craig, A. D. (2003). Interoception: The sense of the physiological condition of the body. *Current Opinion in Neurobiology, 13*(4), 500–505.

Craig, A. D. (2010). The sentient self. *Brain Structure and Function, 214*(5–6), 563–577.

D'Andrea, W., Ford, J., Stolbach, B., Spinazzola, J., & van der Kolk, B. A. (2012). Understanding interpersonal trauma in children: Why we need a developmentally appropriate trauma diagnosis. *American Journal of Orthopsychiatry, 82*(2), 187–200.

Davidson, R., & Kabat-Zinn, J. (2003). Alterations in brain and immune function produced by mindfulness meditation. *Psychosomatic Medicine, 65*(4), 564–570.

Davidson, R., & McEwen, B. (2012). Social influences on neuroplasticity: Stress and interventions to promote well-being. *Nature Neuroscience, 15*(5), 689–695.

Davy, C., Dobson, A., et al. (2012). *The Middle East area of operations (MEAO) health study: Prospective study report*. University of Queensland, Centre for Military and Veterans Health, Brisbane, Australia.

Dozier, M., Peloso, E., Lindhiem, O., et al. (2006). Developing evidence-based interventions for foster children: An example of a randomized clinical trial with infants and toddlers. *Journal of Social Issues, 62*(4), 765–783.

Dube, S. R., Felitti, V. J., Dong, M., Chapman, D. P., Giles, W. H., & Anda, R. F. (2003). Childhood abuse, neglect and household dysfunction and the risk of illicit drug use: The Adverse Childhood Experiences study. *Pediatrics, 111*(3), 564–572.

Farhi, D. (1996). *The breathing book*. New York, NY: Owl.

Feldman, R., Eidelmann, A., Sirota, L., & Weller A. (2002). Comparison of skin-to-skin (kangaroo) and traditional care: Parenting outcomes and preterm infant development. *Pediatrics, 110*(1), 16–26.

Feuerstein, G. (1998). *The yoga tradition: Its history, literature, philosophy, and practice*. Prescott, AZ: Hohm.

Ford, J., Grasso, D., et al. (2013). Clinical significance of a proposed developmental trauma disorder diagnosis: Results of an international survey of clinicians. *Journal of Clinical Psychiatry, 74*(8), 841–849.

Fowler, C. (2002). Review of the book *Visceral Sensory Neuroscience: Interoception. Brain, 126*(6), 1505–1506.

Herman, J. (1992). *Trauma and recovery: The aftermath of violence—from domestic abuse to political terror.* New York, NY: Basic Books.

Herringa, R., Phillips, M., Insana, S., & Germain, A. (2012). Post-traumatic stress symptoms correlate with smaller subgenual cingulate, caudate, and insula volumes in unmedicated combat veterans. *Psychiatry Research, 203*(2–3), 139–145.

Holzel, B. K., Carmody, J., Congleton, C., Yerramsetti, S. M., Gard, T., & Lazar, S. W. (2011). Mindfulness practices leads to increases in regional brain gray matter density. *Psychiatry Research: Neuroimaging Journal, 191*(1), 36–43.

Hrynchak, D., & Fouts, G. (1998). Perception of affect attunement by adolescents. *Journal of Adolescence, 21*(1), 43–48.

International Society for the Study of Trauma and Dissociation. (2011). Guidelines for Treating Dissociative Identity Disorder in Adults, Third Revision. *Journal of Trauma and Dissociation, 12*(2), 115–187.

Kabat-Zinn, J. (1994). *Wherever you go, there you are: Mindfulness meditation.* New York, NY: Hyperion.

Karen, R. (1998). *Becoming attached: First relationships and how they shape our capacity to love.* New York, NY: Oxford University Press.

Khalsa, S., Rudrauf, D., Feinstein, J., & Tranel, D. (2009). The pathways of interoceptive awareness. *Natural Neuroscience, 12*(12), 1494–1496.

Khoury, L., Tang, Y., Bradley, B., Cubells, J., & Ressler, K. (2010). Substance use, childhood traumatic experience, and posttraumatic stress disorder in urban civilian population. *Depression and Anxiety, 27*(12), 1077–1086.

Kinniburgh, K., Blaustein, M., & Spinazzola, J. (2005). Attachment, self-regulation, and competency: A comprehensive intervention framework for children with complex trauma. *Psychiatric Annals, 35*(5), 424–430.

Krakow, B. et al. (2001). The relationship of sleep quality and posttraumatic stress to potential sleep disorders in sexual assault survivors with nightmares, insomnia, and PTSD. *Journal of Traumatic Stress*, *14*(4), 647–665.

Kurtz, R. (1990). *Body-centered psychotherapy*. Boulder, CO: LifeRhythm.

Lanius, R. A., Williamson, P., Densmore, M., et al. (2001). Neural correlates of traumatic memories in posttraumatic stress disorder: A functional MRI investigation. *American Journal of Psychiatry, 158,* 1920–1922.

Lazar, S., Kerr, C., et al (2005). Meditation experience is associated with increased cortical thickness. *Neuroreport, 16*(17), 1893–1897.

Levine, P. (1997). *Waking the tiger: Healing trauma*. Berkeley, CA: North Atlantic.

Loewenstein, R. J. (2006). DID 101: a hands-on clinical guide to the stabilization phase of dissociative identity disorder treatment. *Psychiatric Clinics of North America, 29,* 305–332.

Long, Z., Duan, X., Xie, B., et al. (2013). Altered brain structural connectivity in post-traumatic stress disorder: A diffusion tensor imaging tractography study. *Journal of Affective Disorders, 150*(3), 798–806.

Lutz, A., McFarlin, D., Perlman, D., Salomons, T., & Davidson, R. (2013). Altered anterior insula activation during anticipation and experience of painful stimuli in expert meditators. *Neuroimage, 64,* 538–546.

Luxenberg, T., Spinazzola, J., & van der Kolk, B. A. (2001). Complex trauma and disorders of extreme stress (DESNOS) diagnosis, part one: Assessment. *Directions in Psychiatry, 21,* 373–392.

Morey, R. A., Petty, C. M., et al. (2008). Neural systems for executive and emotional processing are modulated by symptoms of posttraumatic stress disorder in Iraq war veterans. *Journal of Psychiatric Research, 162*(1), 59–72.

Morey, R. A., Dolcos, F., et al. (2009). The role of trauma-related distractors on neural systems for working memory and emotion processing in posttraumatic stress disorder. *Journal of Psychiatric Research, 43*(8), 809–817.

Ogden, P., Minton, K., & Pain, C. (2006). *Trauma and the body*. New York, NY: W. W. Norton.

Rhodes, A.M. (2014). Yoga for traumatic stress (Dissertation: Boston College).

Rothschild, B. (2000). *The body remembers.* New York, NY: W. W. Norton.

Samuelson, K. (2011). Post-traumatic stress disorder and declarative memory functioning: A review. *Dialogues in Clinical Neuroscience, 13*(3), 346–351.

Saper, C., Scammell, T., & Lu, J. (2005). Hypothalamic regulation of sleep and circadian rhythms. *Nature, 437*(7063), 1257–1263.

Shapiro, F. (2001). *Eye movement desensitization and reprocessing (EMDR): Basic principles, protocol, and procedures* (2nd ed.). New York, NY: Guilford Press.

Sharafkhaneh, M. D., et al. (2005). Association of psychiatric disorders and sleep apnea in large cohort. *SLEEP, 28*(11), 1405–1411.

Spinazzola, J., Habib, M., et al. (2013). The heart of the matter: Complex trauma in child welfare. *CW360° Trauma-Informed Child Welfare Practice,* Winter 2013, University of Minnesota.

Steele, K., van der Hart, O., & Nijenhuis, E.R.S. (2005). Phase-oriented treatment of structural dissociation in complex traumatization: Overcoming trauma-related phobias. *Journal of Trauma & Dissociation, 6*(3), 11–53.

Stern, D. (1985). *The interpersonal world of the infant.* New York, NY: Basic Books.

Terr, L. (1992). *Too scared to cry.* New York, NY: Basic Books.

Tick, E. (2005). *War and the soul.* Wheaton, IL: Quest Books.

van der Kolk, B. A. (1994). The body keeps the score. *Harvard Review of Psychiatry, 1,* 253–265.

van der Kolk, B. A. (2006). Clinical implications of neuroscience research. *Annals of the New York Academy of Science, 1071,* 277–293.

van der Kolk, B., Stone, L., West, J., Rhodes, A., Emerson, D., Suvak, M., & Spinazzola, J. (2014). Yoga as an Adjunctive Treatment for Posttraumatic Stress Disorder: A Randomized Controlled Trial. *Journal of Clinical Psychiatry, 75*(0)

West, J. (2011). Moving to heal: Women's experience of therapeutic yoga after complex trauma. PhD dissertation, Boston College.

Wurmser, L., & Jarass, H. (2013). Introduction. In L. Wurmser & H. Jarass (Eds.), Nothing good is allowed to stand: An integrative view of the negative therapeutic reaction (pp. 1–25). New York: Routledge.

Yates, T. (2004). The developmental psychopathology of self-injurious behavior: Compensatory regulation in posttraumatic adaptation. *Clinical Psychology Review, 24*, 35–74.

Yehuda, Daskalakis, Lehrner, Desarnaud, Bader, Makotkine, Flory, Bierer, and Meaney (2014). Influences of maternal and paternal PTSD on epigenetic regulation of the glucocorticoid receptor gene in holocaust survivor offspring. *American Journal of Psychiatry, 171*, 872–880.

Yehuda, R., et al. (1995). Learning and memory in combat veterans with posttraumatic stress disorder. *American Journal of Psychiatry, 152*(1), 137–139.

# INDEX

action
  clinical meaning of, 81
  definition of, 81
  purpose and, 114–117
  *see also* taking action
Adverse Childhood Experiences,
    25, 31–32
afferent nervous system, 44
Ainsworth, M., 24, 25
anterior cingulate cortex, 22, 23
attachment theory, 24–28, 31
  implications for treatment,
    32–34, 35
attunement, 148–150
avoidance, 136–137

Back and Shoulder Stretch, 159,
    160
being present
  as body experience, 95, 103
  clinical significance of, in TSY,
    99–100
  creating opportunity for, 108
  definition of, 105
  evolution of clinical conceptu-
    alization of, 95–100
  feet on floor exercise to pro-
    mote, 94–95, 104–106
  interoception and, 103–105

meaning of, 100–102
trauma as barrier to, 99,
    102–103
TSY practices to promote, 105–
    108, 175
Bowlby, J., 25, 35
breathing
  awareness of movement in,
    125–126
  current understanding of
    trauma effects on, 121–122
  exercise to invite awareness of,
    124–125
  inviting clients to deepen,
    126–127
  long out breath, 6–7
  in mainstream yoga, 2–3
  nasal, 127–128
  practices to promote dynamic
    experiencing of, 123–124
  therapeutic goals in work with,
    123
  in TSY, 6–7, 121, 122–123
Broca's area, 23

chair-based yoga, 109–111
choice
  adaptive response to trauma
    perceived as, 64–66

trauma experience (*continued*)
  attachment theory and, 24–28
  avoiding coercive communication in, 52–54
  compared with other somatic interventions, 10–14
  connection between emotion and body experience in, 13–14
  distinguishing features of, as yoga practice, 3
  empowerment goals in, 20–21
  facilitator's language in, 8–10, 67–69
  focus on present moment in, 90
  indication for, 37–38
  integration of foundational principles for change in, 87–90
  mechanism of change in, 32, 55–56, 86–87
  neural changes associated with, 24
  practice examples and case vignettes, 41–43, 59–61, 79–80, 93–94, 109–111, 131–135, 138–139, 140–141
  prohibition against physical contact with client in, 73–77

  theory of trauma in, 14–21, 31–34
  use of forms in, 3–6
  use of mindfulness in, 8
trauma treatment
  benefits of empowerment in, 66–67
  current somatic models for, 10–14
  relational nature of, 144
  self-regulation goals in, 56–58
  *see also* trauma-sensitive yoga (TSY)
TSY. *see* trauma-sensitive yoga

van der Kolk, B., 21, 23, 89, 99, 104, 116, 137
visceral experience, 44–47

war veterans, 37–38

Yehuda, R., 98
yoga
  common features of practices in, 2–3
  poses in, 3–4
  TSY and, 3
  *see also* trauma-sensitive yoga (TSY)